The Way
to Go

The Way to Go

PORTRAIT OF A
RESIDENTIAL HOSPICE

Marietta Pritchard

NORTHAMPTON, MASSACHUSETTS

The Way to Go is published by
The Impress Group,
Northampton, Massachusetts.
Text copyright ©2015 by Marietta Pritchard
All rights reserved

ISBN # 978-1-4951-4011-2

Cover photograph by Carol Lollis
Photographs copyright ©2015 by Carol Lollis

PRINTED IN THE UNITED STATES

Be careful, then, and be gentle about death.
For it is hard to die, it is difficult to go through
the door, even when it opens.

—D. H. Lawrence, from "All Souls' Day"

CONTENTS

Author's Note

THE STAFF OF THE FISHER HOME have been unfailingly helpful as I gathered information and impressions for this book. This has also been true of the families that I spoke with. I am grateful for their openness and trust. Although it will be clear to the reader that I have great admiration for this organization, this is in no way an officially sanctioned or commissioned piece of writing. It is not a marketing tool, but a work of journalism. Needless to say, the book's flaws are all mine.

Throughout the book, I have used real names wherever the people interviewed have understood that that would be the case. In my journal excerpts, which appear here and there in the book, I have mostly used initial letters—and not the person's real initials.

One caveat: Like all vital organizations, the Fisher Home is a work in progress, a moving target for a writer. Since I finished this book in 2013, there have been changes in staff, none of which have altered the overall goals or character of the hospice.

ALPHABETICAL LIST OF FISHER HOME STAFF MENTIONED IN *THE WAY TO GO*

Beth Bachand – Certified Nursing Assistant (CNA)

Paul Berman, M.D. – Medical Director

Mark Bigda, M.D. – Medical Director

June Bishop – CNA

Kathy Curtis – Registered Nurse (RN), Clinical Director

Matt DeLuca – RN

Ali Diamond – Manager of the Hospice Shop

Lucy Fandel – RN

Karen Howery – Administrative Assistant

Sharon Kemp – CNA

Margot Menkel – CNA

Jenn Messinger – CNA, and team leader of CNAs

Ilsa Myers – Volunteer Coordinator

Bob Nelson – RN

Norma Palazzo – Spiritual and Bereavement Counselor

Cheryl Poulin – CNA

Maria Rivera – Community Nurse

Donna Sarro – Business Manager

Maxine Stein – Executive Director

Monica Susskind – Community Nurse

Priscilla White – Social Worker

Good Endings

I N RECENT YEARS, our local newspaper has stopped having staff members write obituaries and has created a kind of do-it-yourself page. Family members or friends write the life story of the person who has just died, with only the slightest editorial help from the newspaper. This makes for noteworthy stylistic variations, from the scrupulously formal to the wildly improvisational, from the drily factual to the warmly emotional. In many cases, however, a formulaic start to the obituary has emerged. The first sentence reads something like this: "Joe Smith, ninety, died peacefully yesterday at his home after a short illness, surrounded by his loving family." That sentence puts in a nutshell what many would call a good death. At ninety, Joe was old enough so that we could say he'd had a good run; the death was peaceful; it happened at home; it was a short illness, so the dying didn't take too long; and the family was present and evidently loving, at least at the end.

It is, perhaps, what we might wish for ourselves, if we've spent any time thinking about it—a good death, short, peaceful, not too painful, at a ripe old age, on good terms with our family members. Along with that, we'd probably also prefer to have what usually doesn't appear in the obituary: all our wits and all our affairs in order—our wills made, the last sentence of our memoir written, that final carpentry project finished, the garden weeded, our bills paid, and our possessions allocated to the people who will want and appreciate them.

IT IS JUST SUCH A GOOD DEATH that the movement and way of thinking known as hospice aims to provide. After many decades of the increasing medicalization and technologizing of death, hospice has fought to restore human and spiritual content to the end of life. It is founded on the conviction that a person's last days can be peaceful, even fulfilling, and need not be accompanied either by pain or by aggressive medical treatment. It emphasizes comfort, quality, and choice at the end of life.

Doctors and nurses working with hospice often need to be re-educated. Their traditions and training impel them to make people better, to cure diseases. These impulses sometimes run counter to the hospice belief that when people are approaching the end of life, the best course is to make them and their families as comfortable as possible, since efforts to cure often cause additional discomfort, both physical and emotional. Few people these days would choose to end life in a hospital, with its emphasis on high-tech treatments, its machines and rigid schedules, its industrial-strength bustle and noise. Hospice aims to bring the dying person to a place where the care is both calm and effective. There is always the hope, too, that given the chance to be free from medical intrusions, the person may find a way to fulfill some important wishes—attend a grandchild's wedding, finish a work of art, enjoy sitting in a favorite sunny spot outdoors.[*]

---

[*] An eloquent book by Dr. Ira Byock, *Dying Well: Peace and Possibilities at the End of Life* (New York: Berkley Publishing Group, 1997), addresses that goal.

Much of the hospice care in this country is delivered in people's homes, where a hospice team provides the services of an aide for up to a few hours a day, a nurse once a week or more, and a social worker and spiritual counselor. Trained volunteers are also available to come to the home to cook meals, keep people company, run errands. Hospice provides what is called "durable medical equipment" such as hospital beds, commodes, and wheelchairs, as well as medication. This lifts a great burden from family and caregivers. But although most people would prefer to die at home, the bulk of care there—twenty or more hours a day—must be borne by the family, their friends, or by hired help.

Not everyone has a home that lends itself to the demanding care so often needed at the end of life. Sometimes caregivers—spouses, children—are worn out from weeks or months of lack of sleep and unrelenting work. Often they are ailing or elderly themselves. Often they don't feel they have the skills or the energy to go on. And there are dying people who do not have families or other caregivers nearby. For all of these people, a residential hospice is an unanticipated gift. The one that is the focus of this book, the Hospice of the Fisher Home in Amherst, Massachusetts, offers both home and residential care, with a smooth transition from hospice services in an individual's home to its hospice residence, where the familiar team is found under a single roof. Care here in the nine-bed residence—physical, emotional, spiritual—takes place twenty-four hours a day, with a registered nurse always on hand and the clinical director and a physician always either present or on call. It is a medically conscientious haven, an oasis for dying people as well as for their families and friends.

&

I HAD BEEN DEEPLY IMPRESSED with the hospice care given in their home to my parents at the end of their lives, and so it didn't take me long to become involved with hospice as a volunteer at the Fisher Home. As I often do with new experiences, I began to keep a journal of my time there. Soon I decided I wanted to share those observations, to try to give the larger world a sense of how this small independent hospice worked. A number of excellent books were available about the theory and practice of hospice, with first-person accounts mostly from professionals, nurses and doctors working in the field. I wanted to do something different: to begin from the standpoint of a journalistic "outsider" and draw a portrait of an extraordinarily humane place and the people who lived and died there, as well as those who worked and volunteered there.

My method has been to observe, talk and listen, and to conduct interviews with staff, families, and, whenever possible, residents. All of these people have been generous with their time and patient with my questions. These conversations and interviews appear as profiles and third-person narratives. They are other people's stories, thoughts, histories. Alternating with these, I have set down excerpts from my own journals, my day-by-day observations as a volunteer, highly subjective and written in the first person. My hope has been to create an inclusive depiction, a mosaic of a complex place and its varied inhabitants, a place that is managing to survive in a world of for-profit medicine while performing the essential work of bringing people through the final passage of their lives in comfort and peace, work that is done gently, cheerfully, and always professionally.

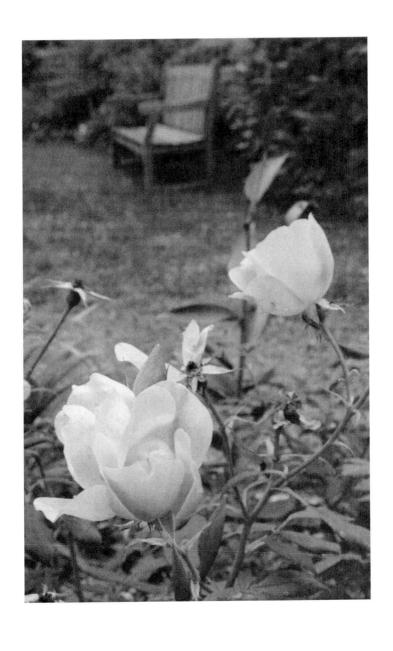

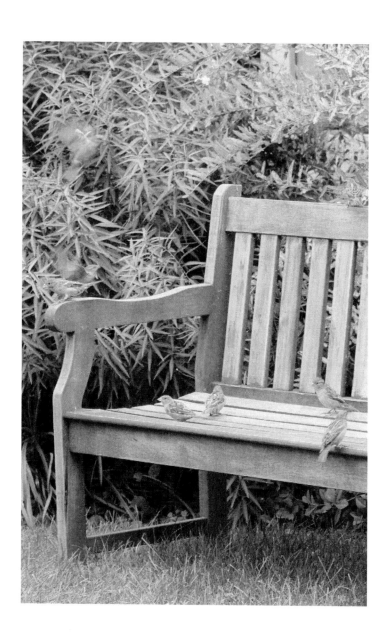

CHAPTER ONE

WHY HOSPICE?

BOTH OF MY PARENTS received hospice care. My father had it back in the late 1980s. Then as now, to be eligible for hospice, the doctor needed to assert that a person suffered from a "life-limiting" condition and had no more than six months to live. My father had had several crises with congestive heart failure, as well as a heart attack. At ninety-two, he was frail and needed oxygen at night. He needed help with bathing, and my mother, who was eighty, was worn out both physically and emotionally. Taking care of sick people had never been her best role. She did it by the book, but with little generosity of spirit.

Now hospice care in their home brought weekly visits from a supervising nurse, but most importantly it brought Jill, a kind and sympathetic home health aide who came to bathe my father several times a week and to see that his oxygen equipment was working properly. My Hungarian-born father became very attached to Jill, which predictably annoyed my Viennese-born mother, who had always been jealous of any woman who was on good terms with her husband—including also her daughters. But Mother eventually learned to be friends with Jill, whom she truly needed.

My father's decline was slow and steady, undramatic despite several brief hospital stays. He was able to read, to communicate fully, to eat and drink, even to go up and down stairs until the last weeks of his life, when he became weak and eventually bedridden. At this point he also stopped eating. Although my sister had come to help out, she was staying with us—Mother's choice—not in our parents' condo, which was only a couple of miles from our house in Amherst. Although Mother was exhausted and more and more worn down emotionally, she never wanted anyone else staying under her roof. Seeing my mother's state, the hospice nurse suggested that our father be taken to the local hospital, where the hospice had several rooms under their charge (there was not yet a residential hospice in the area). My mother tearfully proposed this to him, even though she had hoped he could stay at home. I heard him say, "Whatever is best for you." He was a courtly man to the end.

An ambulance came, and the crew gently carried him out. We followed in our car, my sister, my mother, and I. At the hospital, we were met by our father's doctor, who said he wanted to do some tests. We were shocked. "No more tests," we told him. "He is now under hospice care." He backed off. The room, as it turned out, was not actually run by hospice; there was a non-hospice patient in it for the first day. The second day, Daddy had the room to himself, and in the late afternoon, with my mother and me there, he died quietly.

I HAD WATCHED OVER MY PARENTS after they moved to Amherst in 1984, but my caretaking role did not expand until after my father's death, in August 1988, when my mother was living alone. Mother was fiercely independent in many ways, extremely needy in others. She had found her way into a new community, meeting people at the nearby health club where she swam every day. She met people through my husband, Bill, and me, although she often disapproved of my women friends, whom she found intelligent but too unconventional, not mannerly enough in ways she insisted upon. Her best contacts were through Amherst College, where she audited courses in art history and European culture, and attended events at the museum, impressing and intimidating various young professors with her erudition. Some of those academics became friends, joining her for tea and highbrow conversation. There were also a few older Central Europeans who entered her social circle, but she was wary of these connections. Just because you were both Austrian didn't mean you were going to enjoy each other's company. In fact, this ostensible bond often meant an even higher, more selective set of standards.

When my parents first arrived in Amherst, Mother was seventy-seven, able to drive and move about with ease. She was a lively presence at the health club, where she held court in the Jacuzzi with a wide array of people. She also held more formal weekly tutorials for a friend and me as we struggled to learn Hungarian. She and I worked for several years on her father's letters from Occupied France, a project that eventually became the core of a book I wrote. Mother translated them in long-hand on yellow lined pads, and I transcribed them to my computer. We talked at length, her steel-trap memory filling in the gaps, identifying people and events from forty years past. Beyond that, she was tireless when it came to culture and socializing. We went to concerts and museums together, occasionally to the movies or to plays nearby. She came to our house for meals and other gatherings. My sister and I took her to New York for her ninetieth birthday and to the "real" theater there.

I had been on call for several years, helping her solve domestic problems. She could never learn to use a TV remote, for instance, and would phone me several times a week to announce that the TV was broken, whereupon I would drive over and reformat the remote. But mostly she was self-sufficient and knew how to get the sort of help she needed for the things she wanted to do. She had lived frugally on Social Security along with the investments she had tended to after my father died, and she could still afford to pay for that help. There was someone who cleaned her house, and someone who could drive her places from time to time.

But her hip began to be a problem, and she needed my help getting to appointments with physical therapists and various more and less traditional medical gurus. Eventually the hip had to be replaced, and I stayed nearby until she was on her own again. She continued to swim until she couldn't safely get into and out of the pool, and she walked outdoors every day, even when she had to use a walker. She got physical therapy and religiously did all the prescribed exercises. But gradually she lost that hard-won mobility because of spinal stenosis and two bad knees, which she now refused to have replaced despite her orthopedist's urging. She was over ninety, too old, she said, to endure another major surgery and its aftermath. So she needed a cane and then a walker, and had to give up her car—a real blow. Stairs became an issue. Would she be able to stay in her condo? It had two sets of stairs, from the main floor up to the bedrooms and down to the finished basement and garage.

Mother looked into moving to the local retirement home, where she would have to give up her treasured privacy, not to mention most of her financial resources. She resisted that solution. She looked at a local assisted living residence, where apartments could be rented rather than bought. It was a spiffy-looking place with lots of light, attractive furnishings, and a pleasant staff, but she was having none of it. We ate what she thought was a very bad lunch there, and she was appalled by the tiny apartments, where there would have been no room even for one season's clothes, much less her books. That residence would also have involved enforced socializing with people, some of whom were on the brink of serious dementia. She decided she would stay at home. We now needed to figure out what adaptations would be needed for her current and future disabilities. Most of all, she was going to need help with those stairs. We decided to install two sets of lifts. They would cost $18,000, but that was obviously less than the $250,000 entry fee at the retirement home or even the $36,000 annual rent at the assisted living place.

These calculations were based on the fact that Mother had no real illness, except—and this was a big exception—arthritis. Her heart and lungs were in good shape and she had no osteoporosis, so that even when she fell, as she increasingly did, it wasn't because a bone had spontaneously broken. But pain and the effect of painkillers, along with a serious late-blooming anemia, took their toll. After a couple of years she needed attention around the clock, and the roster of freelancers that

I was then managing was no longer sufficient. Our doctor gave me the name of a nurse who ran her own home care agency. "She's a good egg," he said, in his typically understated way. Deb Patulak turned out to be a godsend, an efficient, smart, competent, incredibly hardworking person who ran a staff of home health aides. She would also make nursing calls when necessary, which eliminated emergency room visits when lesser crises occurred, as they more frequently did.

But there came a time when Deb's staff had reached their limits. We needed a hospital bed, a commode, and regular nursing visits. Pain medication needed closer monitoring. The physical and medical demands of Mother's care had now been ramped way up. And so, on the recommendation of our doctor, we called in hospice. They had cared for my father in his last days in the same condo where Mother still lived, and we trusted them.

Hospice is a wonderful organization, but it doesn't always seem that way to those who are about to enter it. "She is very stupid," my mother said, in her best dismissive Viennese tone, about the hospice nurse who had just interviewed her. The woman was young, a little stiff, and very much playing by the rules. She was not dressed in anything a ninety-six-year-old would recognize as nurse's garb, but in bleached denim overalls with a colored T-shirt underneath. Not unusual attire in our culturally diverse, laid-back part of the world, but not the kind of professional appearance Mother expected. This was a somber moment for us all, and it deserved the trappings of respect. Mother was being asked—no, told—to accept the fact that death was near and that although she would always be kept comfortable, further efforts to control her anemia would be discontinued. The nurse was not stupid, only awkward. My mother was attempting to shoot the messenger.

She did, however, eventually get the message. One day a few weeks after hospice took over her care, when she was bedridden, attached to a urinary catheter, and eating almost nothing, she asked me straight out: "Am I dying?" I gulped, wanting to avoid the answer, but had earlier gotten some good help from an older nurse. Yes, I said, and we are going to miss you. My mother seemed relieved. She died about a week later, on December 9, 2003, not exactly peacefully—that was not her way—but with some degree of acceptance. Hospice had made things easier for both of us.

THREE YEARS LATER, I learned that the Fisher Home, a residential hospice with six beds, was about to open in Amherst. It was good news. Many people, my father among them, could have benefitted from having hospice care delivered in just such a homelike setting, thus sparing my mother the exhausting care of his last months. I spotted a newspaper notice announcing that this place would be looking for volunteers. I didn't know what a hospice volunteer did, but I had done other kinds of service over the years—tutoring high school kids, teaching English as a second language to adults, editing publications for nonprofits. I clipped the notice and kept it on my desk for a few months, picking it up and looking at it from time to time. I came to realize that after attending to my parents in their latter days, I was missing contact with people in that final chapter of life. I phoned and signed up. A six-week training course provided a grounding in hospice principles and in what is expected of volunteers. In June 2007, I began my regular twice-weekly visits to the hospice.

HOSPICE HAS EXISTED in some form for centuries. In the Middle Ages in Europe, a hospice was a place of shelter, often a monastery, where weary travelers could stop and where, if they were ill, they could be cared for. But hospice as we now know it, with its trained medical staff and a team of caring professionals, came into being in 1967 in London, when Cicely Saunders (later Dame Cicely) founded St. Christopher's Hospice. St. Christopher's was and is a residential center—now a group of facilities—devoted to the physical, social, psychological, and spiritual needs of the dying and their families. It was the first research and teaching hospice linked with clinical care, and sparked a movement in Great Britain toward the development of similar programs. Two years later, Elisabeth Kübler-Ross published her hugely influential book *On Death and Dying.* Five years later, in 1974, the Connecticut Hospice in Branford opened, the first residential hospice in the United States.

Saunders' concern was that sound medical practice should be combined with the expertise of a team attending to a dying person's spiritual, emotional, and practical concerns. Sympathy and tender loving care were important but by no means sufficient, and she studiously avoided sentimentalizing what she was trying to do. First-class medicine came first, with control of pain and other symptoms. As she wrote: "A patient, wherever he may be, should expect the same analytical attention to terminal suffering as he received for the original diagnosis and treatment of his condition. The aim is no longer cure, but the chance of living to his fullest potential in physical ease and activity and with the assurance of personal relationships until he dies."* In the hospice movement, she said, "we continue to be concerned both with the sophisticated science of our treatments and with the art of our caring, bringing competence alongside compassion."†

THE HOSPICE MOVEMENT'S CONCERNS about pain control and individual autonomy at the end of life have striking parallels with those surrounding the natural childbirth movement. That movement,

---

* Cicely Saunders and Mary Baines, *Living With Dying* (Oxford: Oxford University Press, 1983), vi.

† Cicely Saunders, "The Founding Philosophy," in Dame Cicely Saunders, Dorothy H. Summers, and Neville Teller, eds, *Hospice: The Living Idea* (Philadelphia: W. B. Saunders, 1981), 4.

which gained strength in the 1970s, along with other "liberation" movements, was an attempt to demedicalize childbirth, educating people to see it as a normal, family-centered process. Anesthesia was reduced and sometimes avoided altogether; husbands and other family and friends were invited into delivery rooms and home births to share in the great event. Something remarkably similar began to happen around the same time about attitudes toward death. Kübler-Ross' book encouraged patients, families, and doctors to look frankly and fearlessly at death and to try to understand the responses of dying people.

Meanwhile, medical technology was becoming increasingly sophisticated. People could be kept "alive" on machines, on artificial hearts, on feeding tubes. Cancer treatments included chemotherapies that often produced devastating side effects, adding days to lives, if not always life to those days. More people died in hospitals, even as hospitals began to be seen as places where no one wanted to die. It was in this climate that the hospice movement began to flourish. Since 1974, with the founding of the Connecticut Hospice, thousands of hospice organizations have come into existence, most of them providing care at home for the dying. In

2012, the U.S. had 5,500 such organizations, serving over a million and a half people. Only a few of them were small, independent, nonprofit enterprises such as the Fisher Home.* Because their labor-intensive services are not fully covered by Medicare or other insurance payments, residential hospices tend to lose money. As a result, most of them survive with the financial support of home hospice and visiting nurses services, and many exist within the physical context of larger hospitals or nursing homes, some of which are for-profit businesses.

Hospice is not primarily a place or a group of people, but rather a set of principles and a course of action embodying a mission. Many organizations in recent years have devised what is known as a mission statement. McDonald's has one and so does Courtyard by Marriott. In these commercial entities the difference between mission statement and reality may not be terribly important to consumers. If the desk clerk is not especially friendly or attentive, you can still have a pretty good night at the Marriott. But for dying people entering hospice care, the promises made by

---

* *NHPCO's Facts and Figures: Hospice Care in America.* (Alexandria, VA: National Hospice and Palliative Care Organization, 2013), 4, 8.

an organization devoted to their comfort are crucial. Hospice says, in effect: "We will work to make your last days not only comfortable but meaningful. We will attend also to the needs of your family during that time, then support them through the weeks and months after your death."

Hospice seeks to normalize death. But for many people in our culture, death is never seen as normal. It is the unspeakable, the word that cannot be uttered except in a hushed whisper, the event that cannot be faced. It is a long way from this avoidance and terror to the peaceful departure that is a hospice goal.

A couple of anecdotes: In the early days of my volunteering, I was having lunch with another hospice volunteer at a small, homestyle restaurant, and we were talking about our experiences, our thoughts about the Fisher Home and the end of life. A woman at a nearby table eating with her daughter got up and came over, visibly upset. "Please talk more quietly," she said. "Oh, sorry," we said. "We didn't realize we were too loud." "No, it's not that," said the woman, "but you were talking about death, and you shouldn't do that in a public place."

Death, to put it in the most banal terms, is definitely a problem, something our culture prefers to sweep under the emotional rug. Poetry, religious hymns, and memorial services are some of the few places it can be spoken of freely. Why, we might ask, is it not a trusted and revered companion, like birth? Why can't we be persuaded that there is a time for all things, a time to live and a time to die, as Ecclesiastes has it? Can we honestly say, as in the Paul Simon tune, "Hello, darkness, my old friend"? Or do we believe that it is more admirable, more heroic, more understandable to struggle, to fight, and not go gentle into that good night—all the while not even talking about it?

Another anecdote: Bill and I were set to have dinner with someone I'll call Larry, a school friend of his in their upstate New York hometown. A smart, quirky guy in his early eighties, Larry was a small-town lawyer who had kept in touch with Bill over the years, and especially through the course of his decades-long treatment for prostate cancer. Larry's cancer had now metastasized. In their letters, the two mainly liked to exchange memories from high school and especially to compete in recalling details about the sports teams Larry had played on and about the bands they'd both played in. But our dinner together was not to be. His wife, Miranda, called: Larry had

had a crisis and was in the hospital. When we visited him there, we learned that his condition was dire. After numerous surgeries and chemotherapies for his cancer, he was now developing blood clots in his bladder that caused him terrible pain. Miranda had been able to handle this at home for a time, but now he needed to be in the hospital.

When we arrived at the big municipal hospital, we found Larry in a small room for two patients with a curtain between them. Miranda was in the crowded hallway talking to a doctor while noisy human traffic swirled around them. She was distraught. Larry had asked her to bring his living will to the hospital, but she was reluctant to do so because she thought it would mean refusing treatment that she still wanted him to have. While I talked with Miranda, who poured out her worries, Bill and Larry had a lively talk—Larry doing most of the talking, as usual—about the past, especially about sports and music. But what he was also saying was that he'd had enough of being treated and being miserable, and wanted now to be allowed to die. This was said several times, loud and clear. What was also clear was that Miranda was not hearing him and that, in spite of how long he had been ill and in spite of how long they had been married, they hadn't really spoken to each other or to any trusted medical person about the end of his life. They had no children and few intimate friends.

She was afraid, among other things, that if he were to come home, he would commit suicide. He had said as much. He was an avid hunter, traveling to Canada with his buddies for elk hunting over the years. He had a large collection of guns—hunting guns in a locked case and handguns in a safe. Miranda told me that she didn't know where he kept the keys to these guns. I took a deep breath and asked whether she had considered hospice care for him. She started back, alarmed, and said, "But that's only for people who are dying!" Right you are, was what I didn't say. I was not her close friend, and it didn't seem my place to point it out. What I did say was that maybe hospice could keep him more comfortable and out of crisis, since he didn't seem to want more treatment. Was there a hospital social worker or someone else she could talk to? She said she would think about it.

The advance of medicine in our time has brought with it a paradox. Instead of dying quickly as our forebears did of infectious diseases, of heart attacks and strokes, we can be rescued from these scourges of the past and kept alive by medication and machines. The result is that more of us will die what Stephen P. Kiernan in his book *Last Rights* calls a slow or gradual death.* And in some cases, we will enter a kind of medical limbo that few people would choose or even describe as living. This was Larry's situation. Most of us, if we had the foresight, would rather not go through long, arduous, and ultimately futile medical treatments at the end of our lives. Yet slow death offers an opportunity, too, if we are lucky enough. Without intense treatment, but with the control of pain and other symptoms, it is just this gradual dying that offers the possibility for what hospice describes as a "good death."

In what I see as the best of all possible worlds, my husband's friend could have benefitted from the ministrations of the Fisher Home's staff, who would have sat down with this couple to learn what their wishes were and to try to help them resolve the conflict we observed. The difference in ambience between that bustling, crowded, impersonal hospital corridor and a quiet room in the hospice residence could not be greater.

---

* Stephen P. Kiernan, *Last Rights: Rescuing the End of Life from the Medical System* (New York: St. Martin's, 2006).

When discord is not resolved, we may see such wrenching legal battles as those that have made headlines in recent years. The Terry Schiavo and Karen Quinlan cases were marked by terrible disagreements about how to treat—or not treat—someone with no chance of recovering any recognizable quality of life. The courts and even Congress got involved, while both women languished for years in what is called a persistent vegetative state. Eventually both were allowed to die, after external respirators and feeding tubes were removed.

Ethical dilemmas surely exist in all aspects of medicine, but they are particularly notable and agonizing at the end of life. Hospice staff and volunteers are educated in hospice principles and are accustomed to thinking about the kind of decision making that may be necessary at such times. But patients and families—like Larry and his wife—often have to take a crash course.

ONE THING I HAVE LEARNED as a hospice volunteer is that people confront death in every possible human way—from anger to sadness to resignation to hopefulness and good humor. The role of the hospice staff and volunteers is to help residents attain the goal of a "good death" in whatever way possible, to make the most of their last days, to live them to the fullest. During their time at the Fisher Home, residents, if they are conscious enough, are able to make their own decisions about how they will spend their time: how much company they want; what foods they do and don't want; what kind of music or TV they want; how much medication for pain or other symptoms they want. The interdisciplinary hospice team meets each week to discuss all residents' conditions and to devise strategies for making their days easier. The process by which people end their lives is often referred to as a journey. With hospice, every effort is made to see that pain and suffering are not constant companions on that road.

It is easy enough to achieve total pain control by deeply sedating a patient. But that may not be the person's choice. Some people choose to experience as little pain as possible, even if this means a loss of alertness. Others prefer to endure some discomfort in order to be awake, to understand and take part in what is going on around them. It is a difficult balancing act to find the right amount of medication to alleviate the effects of disease yet not knock people out or flood them with unpleasant side effects. This balancing act goes on all the time in the Fisher Home, where the staff has the services not only of the house doctor but of a pain specialist, who helps devise strategies, both medical and nonmedical, to control people's symptoms.

Most of the Fisher Home staff see their work there as more than a job. It is, rather, a vocation, a calling. A number of the staff have had wide-ranging experience that has brought them to this work relatively late in life. Almost all of those who stay in hospice work say they cannot imagine working anywhere else. It is special, meaningful. More than one describes it as comparable to helping people give birth—the passage at the other end of life, and equally important.

ಎ

BILL CALLS VOLUNTEERING at the hospice my job, but there's a big difference. I've had jobs, and they come with clear responsibilities. Although it's true that I've committed to two-hour visits twice a week, the nice thing about volunteering at the hospice is that you make it up as you go along. That may feel like work at times—cooking, folding laundry, stuffing envelopes, being a hostess to visitors, trying to make residents more comfortable. But it's also something like being a visiting grandmother: When there's a situation you can't or shouldn't handle, you can always call in the people who are really responsible.

At the Fisher Home there are about fifty volunteers, most of whom come for one or sometimes two two-hour shifts a week. Volunteers don't deal with people's bodily functions. The closest thing to this might be helping feed people who can't manage it themselves. But there are plenty of chances to provide company, both spoken and silent, to residents as well as their families. In terms of human contact, you encounter a rich mix. Some people arrive in full possession of their wits, wanting to talk about politics and books, about their families, their hobbies, their work, their lives. They need conversation, to look forward and backward, to complain about the food and the staff, to praise the food and the staff. Sometimes they want to talk about the end of their lives and to try to finish personal business with families and friends. Sometimes they want to read and be read to, to make and listen to music. Sometimes they just want to be left alone with their thoughts.

Other people arrive with their bodies declining but their minds even more deeply impaired. They may be confused or angry or simply withdrawn. They may or may not want company, or they may just want someone to sit quietly with them or take them outdoors in a wheelchair on a nice day.

Then there is a third category, those who arrive at the hospice in the very final stages of their lives, physically depleted, sometimes comatose. Being with these people is essentially a vigil, with quiet talk or singing and some gentle physical contact—stroking an arm or a forehead—or just silent sitting.

For me, this work is tremendously satisfying. In one way you might say it helps me put my own troubles into perspective, but that doesn't fully account for the satisfaction. There is a kind of meditative quality to the experience, despite the fact that it's often so down-to-earth and sometimes even hectic, as it is in any home where there are a lot of visitors. But just as importantly, there is also the possibility of making a small difference in the life of someone who doesn't have a lot of it left. For me, at seventy-seven, with more time behind me than ahead, this naturally means I am looking at my own life and trying to imagine myself and my family in similar situations.

At the start of our volunteer training, we were

asked why we thought we wanted to spend time at the hospice. Many people had a personal connection, as was true for me—a relative or friend had had hospice care and it had impressed them. But one of the women gave a surprising response: "My book group suggested that I become a volunteer because I'm so afraid of death." This certainly seemed counterintuitive to me. She completed the volunteer training, but in the end never came into direct contact with dying residents, choosing instead to become the weekly grocery shopper. She and her husband would arrive with bags of food and cans and boxes and paper products, deposit them in the kitchen, and leave. It worked for her—a perfectly legitimate way of helping out without having to confront her fears directly.

Her response has made me wonder: Do I confront my own fears there? Or do I just escape the ordinary wear and tear of my life by immersing myself in other people's needs? Hard to say. I'm certainly less afraid of death now than I was as a child. It is the lead-up to death that frightens me, if it means debility, loss of mental capacity, loss of self, physical pain, spiritual distress, or fear itself. These troubles can be alleviated in a well-run hospice. Death itself, the "distinguished thing," in Henry James' words—this does not terrify me. I do not posit an afterlife, except in the form of compost or in the memories of others, aided in my case, perhaps, by words on the page. My time is now.

But that still doesn't answer the question of what volunteering at a hospice does for me. In the absence of "real" work, it provides an anchor to my week, which is otherwise filled with many things, including the increasing amount of personal maintenance that aging demands. It provides, too, I realize, the kind of colleagues that I have missed since I left my job as an editor at the local newspaper. These are the people you work with, with whom you have regular contact, but who are not the same as your friends and family. They may become friends and then exist outside the work setting, but the relationship within the workaday world is no less genuine. With friends, you have each other's lives to talk about, each other's woes and pleasures to share. You have deep confidences—relationships that can bring both joys and disappointments. Friends need to be, as the cliché has it, "there for you." With colleagues, you may share confidences but rarely intimacy. This is a nice difference. You leave your work and your colleagues at the workplace.

At the hospice, my colleagues include the aides, who do the heavy lifting. They handle the residents' personal care, bathing them, transferring them from bed to wheelchair, from wheelchair to toilet, changing their incontinence briefs, emptying their bedpans and catheter bags. They cook and deliver meals, and often establish relationships with residents and their families. I can help with some of these things—not personal care, but cooking, kitchen cleanup, delivering meals, folding laundry, taking out trash. Because I have no fixed job description, I can take my time with the residents as aides cannot—sitting and talking with people while they eat, joining them in watching TV, or reading to them. I spend time listening to families and learning about their worries, their lives, their relationships. And as I work alongside the aides, cooking or doing dishes, I learn about their concerns, too, their families, their hopes and dreams.

My colleagues are also the nurses, who are responsible for all of the medical care. From them, I've learned something about the complexity of caring for people in their final days. Of course I take on none of the nursing tasks, but I can sometimes lighten the load by providing a resident with distraction or company, by talking with families, by answering phones or call bells.

In addition I count as colleagues the five women who manage the place: the volunteer coordinator, the social worker, the spiritual counselor, the clinical director, and the executive director. These are the people who look out for the physical, social, psychological, and spiritual care of residents, families, and the hospice staff, and who keep the place on an even keel financially and physically, and in good compliance with the constantly shifting maze of Medicare and state health regulations. They are often concerned with basic practicalities—how to get the grocery shopping and food preparation done efficiently; how to get a computer set up; how to see that someone gets a chair that is comfortable; how to get a resident to her grandson's graduation safely. Their official jobs are overseeing the clinical and business aspects of the hospice, coordinating the volunteers, making sure that families get the psychological and spiritual support they need, addressing matters of belief and bereavement—and above all, doing this in a medically responsible and appropriate way. We volunteers fill in the gaps when and as we can.

Yet there certainly is a way in which volunteering at a hospice keeps me from forgetting that life ends (not that, in my eighth decade, I need too much reminding). What working in a hospice also teaches me is that life goes on until its end, and that the last stretch can be as valuable and satisfying as any other part of our existence, if we will allow it to happen that way. Given the choice, I know that like most people, I would want to die at home, under ideal circumstances, under the Fisher Home's home hospice care. But if that turns out not to be possible, then this place, the Fisher Home residence, is what I would choose for myself— the way to go.

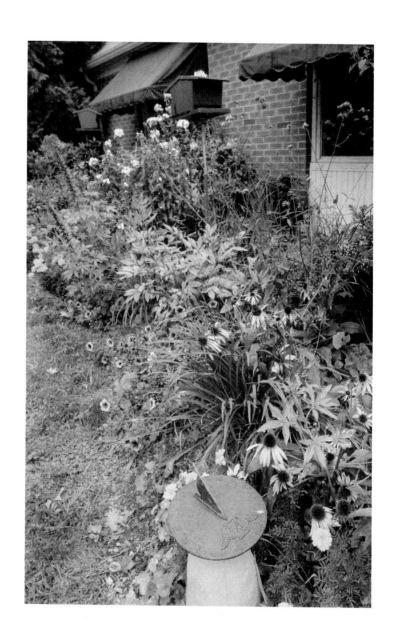

CHAPTER TWO

THE FISHER HOME:
SOME HISTORY

T HE HOSPICE OF THE FISHER HOME opened in November 2006. A former group residence—the Amherst Home for Aged Women—it is a long, low, unobtrusive Colonial-style building, with extensive lawns, ornamental fruit trees, perennial gardens, and a gazebo, set far back from a well-traveled local road. In 2010, a new wing was added containing three additional residents' rooms, bringing the capacity up to nine. Residents have single rooms, some with private baths, some shared with an adjoining room. The spaces are homey, with pictures on the walls, a variety of old-style furniture, colorful hand-made quilts on the beds, and, if wanted, television sets. Residents look out on greenery and bird feeders, and can bring as many of their own possessions as they like—clothing, family photos, favorite paintings and artworks, CD players. A few have brought beloved cats, and one resident acquired a cockatiel. Sometimes people are well enough to use their computers to continue work on unfinished projects or keep in e-mail touch with friends.

The new wing has a sleek, modern look softened by wall hangings and comfortable seating in the hallways. The older part of the building needs no such softening. The living room has an array of upholstered furniture, a small piano, a big TV, houseplants, and lots of natural light. The dining room retains some of the formality of its previous incarnation as a home for elderly ladies, with a brass chandelier above a long dining table, and a cabinet displaying ornate china and glass. The flowered wallpaper might have been found in someone's grandmother's house. The whole place, as many residents and families have noted, feels like a hospitable private home.

In this building, visitors and family are made to feel cared-for. Staff and volunteers keep an eye out for people's needs. Coffee and snacks are available on the kitchen counter; toys and games are there for smaller and larger children; cots can be set up for family members who wish to stay overnight. The building and grounds make it possible for people to have company or privacy as they wish. Amherst has restaurants, walking trails, a movie theater, shops, and a public library within easy reach for visitors who need a break. A bed-and-breakfast across the street offers pleasant quarters for out-of-towners.

IN THE WINTER OF 2000, Northampton resident and retired speech and language therapist Barbara Snoek became convinced that, although a county-wide home hospice organization was already in existence, the community needed something more—a residence to provide hospice services for dying people who could not be cared for at home. The impulse was personal and immediate: Her husband, Diedrick, had had a stroke in June 1995, a year after retiring from Smith College as a professor of psychology. He was sixty-four. Six months after the stroke, he was diagnosed with prostate cancer. Barbara worried about her husband's health, but also about what it would mean for her if he became terminally ill. "She was very open about that," says Diedrick, who is now in good health. "She said, 'I want to be your wife, not your caregiver.'" Moved by her reading of Dr. Ira Byock's book *Dying Well*, which describes the benefits of hospice care, Barbara began to marshal local forces that could make real her vision of a residential hospice. The Friends of Hospice was formed, and the group began to meet regularly, visiting residential hospices in the region, meeting with local hospital officials, exploring grant possibilities.

Early in the process, Barbara contacted Joan Keochakian (Mrs. Hospice, as Diedrick calls her), the founder of home hospice care—Hospice of Hampshire County—in the Pioneer Valley in 1978, almost twenty years earlier. When Barbara described her hopes, Joan exclaimed delightedly, "Where have you been all my life?"

In the meantime, Diedrick turned out not to need any caregiving. "I popped out and recovered," he says. But Barbara was not backing away from her mission. Diedrick adds, "We Quakers say that she had a 'leading.' Something about the Byock book told her: 'This is what I have to do.' "

Then, along with hard work on the part of a number of interested people, came what Diedrick refers to as their three miracles. The first was a state grant. In April 2001, Diedrick had a phone call from a former student who said, "Do you know that the state is giving away leftover money, $8 million from the tobacco settlement? It needs to be for something that benefits elders." They didn't know, but with two weeks left to submit proposals, they went right to work, and delivered their request for $1 million to launch a residential hospice to the state office on the last possible day. "Next thing we know," says Diedrick, still shaking his head in wonder, "they awarded us $485,000, no strings attached."

Hampshire Care, a nursing home just west of Northampton, had offered free land to build on, and an architect drew up plans. But the site occupied a steep hill, and a lengthy sewer line would need to be replaced; the grant money could not cover both the building and the infrastructure changes. Further, there was an even more crucial question: Could the nursing staff of Hampshire Care quickly become a hospice staff? This seemed unlikely, since hospice requires very different training and different attitudes from those that prevail in a nursing home. With so many obstacles, that version of their vision faded.

Meanwhile, another miracle was taking shape. The Amherst Home for Aged Women at the north end of town, also known as the Fisher Home, was in serious decline. Founded in 1906 as a charitable home for needy women, the current structure was built in 1969, and from then on residents paid room and board. But now other retirement options were becoming more attractive, and the home couldn't find enough residents to remain financially viable. Too much money was going to upkeep, plowing the long driveway in winter, and maintaining the building and its extensive grounds. In 2004, its board initiated a conversation with Joan Keochakian. Although the will stipulated that the home should house only women, Joan had several years earlier arranged for a male client of hers who needed hospice care to be housed there. A legal path for housing both men and women had thus been laid down. She had also made the case for adding hospice care as a permanent part of their services. Her connection paid off, and the home's board gave the Friends of Hospice the property and the endowment.

On September 13, 2004, Barbara wrote an ecstatic letter to the Friends:

> After months of discussion, we can now share our good news with you: Effective August 11, the Friends of Hospice House has been gifted with a lovely well-maintained residence which exceeds our dreams! The single-story brick house includes six individually furnished single bedrooms that are combined with semi-private baths. A cozy living room adjoins a generous dining room. There is a professional kitchen

and fully equipped laundry. Special places are the well-appointed library and a gazebo. Bird houses are posted outside every window. The whole is surrounded by lovely grounds, and there is a bus stop outside the door. . . . As you know, "it takes a village to raise a child," and this Residence can be seen as our community child.

Then came the third miracle. The Fisher Home already had a group home license, and the Friends assumed that a hospice in that building would be able to continue to operate as a group home. Although it was an unusual format, they applied to reinstate the license anyway. The Boston authorities turned them down. But, recalls Diedrick, "our lawyer said, 'Let's not get antsy.'" They would go and find out what the obstacle was. He pauses and smiles as he remembers the sequence of events. "So here's the miracle: It snows. It's not bad enough to keep us from getting to Boston, but bad enough so that the director of Elder Affairs—the one who said no—isn't coming in to the office. We talk with two other staff people, one of whom is a lawyer who used to be a hospice nurse and who helps us reframe our application. What we need is a license to operate a community hospice service, and, incidentally, we are located in a house where we can also take in patients." In effect, they created a new model for operating a community hospice service that happens also to have a residence.

Though they now had a license, the Fisher Home still had to meet crucial state and federal requirements to be eligible for Medicare and other forms of insurance. They needed an interdisciplinary team that included a medical director, registered nurses, certified nurses' aides, a social worker, spiritual counselor, and bereavement caregiver. There would be inspections, and the home would be strictly regulated on the handling of drugs. In addition, federal guidelines stipulated that 5 percent of overall care hours needed to come from volunteers. There was a lot of work to be done before the new enterprise could begin its work. Barbara and Diedrick Snoek were on the new board, and they also became volunteers, keeping their hands in the day-to-day operation as soon as the hospice opened in 2006. But in a cruel turn of fate, Barbara, who had been the visionary and founding spirit of the place, died almost without warning of cardiac arrest at the couple's Maine vacation home in October 2010. She was seventy-seven.

DESPITE THE AUSPICIOUS TURNS of events that led to the founding of the Hospice of the Fisher Home, there were plenty of bumps in the road ahead. Soon after its opening, much of the clinical staff resigned in protest over the departure of the clinical director, whom they felt had been treated unfairly. There was also dissatisfaction at the perceived nepotism in the naming of Joan Keochakian's son, Greg, to replace his mother as director. In addition, a state inspection had found some minor irregularities, although no patient had suffered ill effects. The irregularities were quickly corrected and new staffing was found, but the attendant publicity was devastating to a new organization hoping to make its reputation in the community. Nevertheless, within a year, after most of the start-up problems had been resolved, it became clear that the Fisher Home was delivering excellent care, and that the residential hospice was providing a high-quality and much-needed service.

In 2010, a building project brought the number of beds up to nine. The new wing was bright and modern, and included solar panels for generating some of the home's electricity. But problems with management remained. In November 2011, Greg Keochakian resigned. The clinical director, Kathy Curtis, stepped in to wear two hats while the board looked for a new director. Through all this, the task of caring for the dying continued uninterrupted. In spite of what often felt like a leadership vacuum, the staff had become a stable, cohesive group, depending on each other for decision making with the support of the hospice's board. They kept each other's spirits and energy up, but most of all they did their work, the work of bringing meaning and comfort to residents' final days.

In January 2013, Maxine Stein took over the position of executive director. A dynamic and focused presence, she immediately began to make changes. The new broom was sweeping clean. First up was a reorganization of the building itself—offices relocated, a couple of new spaces created out of underused areas. At the same time, Maxine was cleaning up communications, making sure that everyone who worked at the hospice knew who they needed to talk to if there was a question or a problem. And she set to work finding a way to make sure the Fisher Home would stay viable financially, working with the board to let the world know that "this gem, this treasure, this incredible resource" existed, and to reach out to the community for support.

Because the hospice depends so much on its "census," the number of patients it serves, the residence has always been on the verge of losing money. Overhead is a constant, and a clinical staff of between thirty-two and forty-two must be paid. (This variation represents the need for per diem staff at times.) In 2012, the budget was $1.65 million, and 2011 tax returns show that expenses exceeded income. As a "community hospice," the Fisher Home is categorized as a home-care entity, and thus receives a lower rate of Medicare reimbursement for medical costs than "inpatient" hospices, which are more like hospitals. The insurance pays the medical part, but families are responsible for room and board, which currently amounts to $375 a day. Some insurances, including long-term care, will contribute toward room and board. Moreover, says business manager Donna Sarro, the organization has historically seen to it that funding is available to subsidize people who cannot pay some or even any of the room and board fees. The aim has always been to turn no one away. Thirty percent of the people who come here, says Donna, get free or subsidized care. About 12 to 15 percent of the home's revenue is budgeted for some sort of financial aid, much of which currently comes from funds raised by the organization's Hospice Shop. The hospice makes every effort to take people, says Donna, "who never even think that they could be here because of their finances, because they've never had a chance to be in a place like this, which is considered private care."

Maxine Stein is clear that the "community" part of this hospice—the at-home care—needs to be expanded, since it is the best way to keep the organization financially stable. A new community care nurse has been hired, and at the same time Maxine has begun putting together marketing efforts to let the public know that the Fisher Home provides not only much-needed residential care for dying people, but that it also offers its services in people's own homes. This is something she will continue to build on for the financial health of the enterprise.

It's been a rough week, with some
drama in my own family, but as I drive
up to the Fisher Home, I feel myself
exhaling at last. I've been volunteering for several years, and it's always
a relief to be here, somewhere I know
I can be useful, where the expectations are high but limited. You can
fail at being a wife and mother, sister, grandmother, and mother-in-law,
but it is hard to fail at being a hospice volunteer. Whatever you give here
is entered on the plus side of the
ledger.

Things are unusually quiet when
I arrive around eleven in the morning.
Several residents have died since
I was here late last week, and
another, a bright, spunky woman with
advanced cerebral palsy, has no longer
been "declining," which makes her no
longer eligible for hospice. (The official term is "hospice-appropriate.")
She has been moved to a nursing home,
where her family hopes physical therapy might restore some use of her
arms. Without much comprehensible
speech, she had been dependent on
pointing to letters on a letter board,
and now she has been deprived of that.
When she arrived at the hospice, she
was not eating and was having trouble

breathing. She was clearly nearing the
end of her life, but the staff found
ways to cheer her up, to alleviate her
shortness of breath and make her more
comfortable. Then, as sometimes happens here, her condition improved.
She has "graduated."

***

Friendly new aide offers me a cookie
just out of the oven, then suggests I
go and sit with B. He is a big guy,
seventy-five, comatose, with oxygen
tubes in his nose and a rather bloody-
looking catheter bag. He'd collapsed
while mowing his lawn. He mostly stays
put, breathing heavily, but occasionally moves a limb and makes groaning
sounds. I pat him on the shoulder,
talk a bit. Nurse comes in and administers pain medication under his
tongue. A CD player in the room. We
listen to snippets of classical music--
a movement of a Mozart piano concerto,
some "Nutcracker"--I've chosen this
over another CD with New Age piano.
He died the following night. Seems I
was sitting a vigil with him.

***

I ask the nurse if there's anything
she'd like me to do, and she directs
me to a new patient, F., in Room 1.
F. is eighty-seven and very weak,
suffering, as the volunteer notebook
tells me, from ovarian cancer, which
has metastasized. She is lying in bed
watching "The Newlywed Game," and she
seems comfortable, if very weak.
I check to see if she'd like anything
to eat or drink. She says no, but
indicates that she'd like company, so
she and I sit and watch together,
laughing at the silliness of the con-
testants. Her husband and daughter
arrive, and we all enjoy a few moments
of this show. I introduce myself to
them and mention that he and I have
met before, that I was a voice student
of his colleague in the UMass music
department. We reminisce a bit about
my former teacher, his old friend. I
ask if he and his daughter would like
anything to eat or drink, then make
my way out.

In the dining room, N., a tiny
sparse-haired former blonde, is sitting at the long table eating lunch,
a few morsels at a time. Her daughter,

the daughter's partner, and their
cocker spaniel have joined N., who had
a stroke at age forty. The daughter
had quit school to take care of her
then, she tells me. Now seventy, N. is
missing an amputated leg and quite a
bit of mental capacity. In serious
physical decline, she has been deemed
hospice-appropriate, yet she is humorous as well as deeply southern in her
manner. Looking out at the new greenery outside, she says, "I love the
spring, I sure do, yes I do." She can
and often does tell her own story.
After growing up in a large hardscrab-
ble Appalachian family, she and a high
school friend decided to leave for
Washington, D.C., to seek their for-
tunes. N.'s fortune turned out to be
a nice Orthodox Jewish businessman,
whom she met while working as a secretary in his firm. She converted from
her original Baptist tradition to
become an observant Jewish wife,
raising their children in that faith,
keeping a kosher kitchen.

Seeing that N. has plenty of company, I go off to visit Gerard Sterling. His dark brown eyes seem even
more luminous than usual this morning.
He has had his hair brushed and is in

bed listening to the radio. Gerard,
who is in his early sixties, has a
brain tumor and does not get up anymore. I praise his appearance, and he
goes through the motions of being
deeply flattered. We have a little flir-
tation going on, and it pleases us
both. A former emergency room physician, he has been solicitous about the
splint I've been wearing on my wrist
since I broke it on the winter's last
slippery patch a few weeks ago. "How
is. . .?" he asks, unable to find the end
of the sentence. "Much better," I tell
him, "and I'm hoping to have this
thing off by the next time I see you."
He is pleased, despite his few words.
"It will be good. . ." he says, and
trails off. I notice that he now has
a bird feeder at his window, which
he's enjoying. "I know a lot about
birds," he says slowly, articulating
clearly. "Oh, what kind of birds have
you seen?" I ask. Pause. "Well. . ." he
says, "there are Italian birds. . . and
Jewish birds." I laugh. "And Indian
birds." Another pause. "And the Indian
birds make a sound like this." He
emits a low, East Indian-inflected
burble. We both laugh.

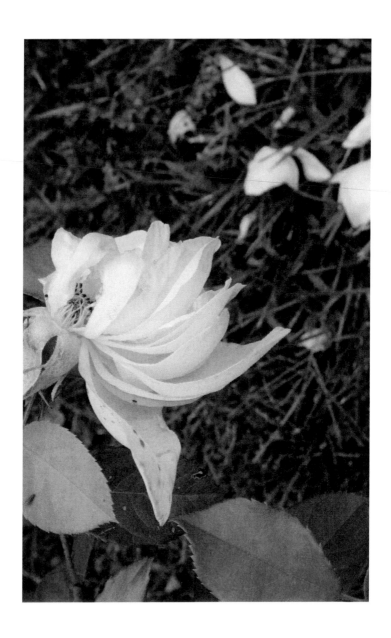

CHAPTER THREE

HOWARD SACHS:
THE STRUGGLE TO ACCEPT

H OWARD SACHS WAS A PROUD MAN, with much to be proud of: proud of the path he had taken from the slums of New York to become a doctor and medical researcher, proud of having brought medical care to the needy in remote and underserved parts of the world, proud of having overcome the effects of a stroke at age sixty-one, proud of his three daughters, Susan, Linda, and Nancy, who admired and loved him. But sharing space with that pride at age eighty-five was a wide streak of anger and bitterness—and he had much to be angry and bitter about. He couldn't forgive or forget the errors of a brain surgeon friend and a neglectful nurse, errors that caused the stroke that derailed his life; and he couldn't stop thinking about a world that treats the elderly and disabled with less than respect. Finally, as painful images rose up to disrupt his final days, he couldn't forgive himself for the deaths he'd caused as a soldier on Okinawa during one of World War II's most terrible battles. At the same time, he was a seeker after spiritual truth, yearning to know whether there is such a thing as a soul, an afterlife, pressing others to be fearless and pursue this search with him.

When he lived in a retirement home in Easthampton, Massachusetts, not far from his daughter Susan, he started a blog, recording his thoughts and memories for several years. Selections from that blog became a memoir, *Skydiving into Medical School*, which he self-published in 2011, just months before his death on December 6 of that year. A nicely produced paperback, the book has many photos of Howard from boyhood through adulthood. The cover image, taken when he was probably in his fifties, shows him literally on top of the world, on a mountain peak somewhere in North America, a romantic hero, slim, fit, with an Abe Lincoln–style beard, hands on hips, looking out over the rugged landscape. By age forty-five he had served in the army, gone to college on the G.I. Bill, married, fathered three children, and divorced his first wife. He became a groundbreaking medical researcher, making crucial discoveries in the field of human hormones. At forty-eight he gave up that prestigious career to enter medical school so that he could work directly with the world's neediest people in Sri Lanka, New Guinea, and other parts of the third world.

When he arrived at the Hospice of the Fisher Home, he was furious. He had severe anemia that he had decided to stop treating with blood and iron transfusions. The anemia, his doctor thought, was caused by an upper gastrointestinal bleed somewhere (which turned out to be the case), but Howard was in no condition to undergo surgery. "That would have killed him," says Susan, "but before it killed him, it would have left him debilitated and in a hospital bed hooked up to a million things—very miserable." Then a badly broken arm from a fall made it impossible for him to use his walker, since the other arm was already out of commission as a result of his stroke. He was becoming malnourished because of the stomach pain he wouldn't tell anyone about. But it was the fall and the break, Susan says, that marked the beginning of the end, precipitating a sharp decline he couldn't bounce back from. Now he was bedridden, entirely dependent on others for his most basic needs. He was angry at the world he had once stood on top of.

Immediately before coming to the Fisher Home, Howard had been in a local nursing home to rehabilitate his arm. Before long he had reached what they thought was his maximum ability to progress, meaning that his insurance would no longer pay for rehab. Susan visited the long-term unit in the same nursing home, where he would have been moved next, "and it was horrible. The only bed they had for him was in a dementia wing, which would have been so cruel, so horrendous for him."

When he came to the hospice, his mind was mostly clear. Unlike many dying people, he had a pretty good idea of what was happening to his body—after all, he was a physician. He knew what would happen next, and was not resigned to it. His own doctor had designated him as eligible for hospice, but Howard was by no means ready to die. On the other hand, Susan was finally able to relax about her father's care. "I loved that place. It was the first time I didn't have to worry about him. He had been in the hospital so many times over the years. He had been in every nursing home in this area, and every time he was in a nursing home or hospital, it was nightmarish, medieval, horrible. I would be so anxious until I could get there and see him."

Susan had been her father's mainstay since 1994, when she had rescued him from a potentially disastrous situation in New Mexico, where he had been living alone and not doing at all well. He was still driving after his stroke, although Susan doesn't know how he managed that, since the stroke had destroyed the left vision field of both eyes. "Can you imagine it? He had no left vision in either eye. He also had what's called left-sided neglect, so that he didn't see things on the left, and he had left-side weakness.

"He called me up from New Mexico one day and said, 'The police are looking for me.' And I said, 'Oh, really? Why?' And he said, 'I don't know.' And I said, 'Well, look, why don't you get on a plane, get out of there, come here, and then I'll find out what's going on.' " She couldn't bear to think of him arrested and in a jail cell. She would get the facts and then, if he had to return to go to court, he would. Susan is a lawyer, practicing in Springfield, Massachusetts. She contacted a lawyer in New Mexico. "It turns out he'd been driving and he'd hit another car and didn't know he had. He hadn't hurt anybody, so it was property damage, hit and run." Eventually the insurance companies all worked it out and that was fine, she says. He didn't get into any legal trouble. "He was here, and he stayed here. I went out to New Mexico and sold his car and closed down his apartment and that was that."

In New Mexico he had been pretty much on his own, having just divorced his second wife, who had taken care of him until then. Says Susan, "He was a very disorganized guy, for all his brilliance, because he always had someone else to do the organizing for him—wives, daughters, lab technicians, postdoctoral students, nurses when he was a doctor. You know, the stuff that women usually handle for men. We do life, we do the details: make sure there's food in the house and the bills are paid. So for a while, my father didn't have anyone doing that for him. I was shocked at his apartment—he was living in squalor. He had one bowl, one fork. I wondered what he'd been eating. The car had a lot of dents in it. I rescued him."

He moved to an apartment in Northampton, where with Susan's assistance and some paid help he was able to manage. Later, there was Susan's assistance and a live-in girlfriend, "unpaid help," as Susan puts it. During that time, he got his Massachusetts medical license and worked in a headache clinic run by a psychologist in Springfield.

Eventually, as his physical condition deteriorated, being on his own was no longer an option, so in March 2004 he moved again, and for seven years lived in the Lathrop retirement community in Easthampton, the town where Susan lives. Life there, as he described it in his blog, was circumscribed and none too happy. He referred to the place as "the morgue." He was proud of the fact that he got outdoors on his walker every morning in all weathers, reminded as he did so of the grand hikes he had taken in the most rugged terrains in the world—the Himalayas and the Amazon basin, among others. The sharp air of a New England winter, despite the treacherous footing for a disabled man, brought him, as he put it, "the sweet breath of life." He expressed deep contempt for those who did not struggle to keep moving as he did, those who merely sat gossiping, waiting for the next meal, waiting for the end. He tried to initiate discussion groups to grapple with big ideas— life, death, the soul—but found little interest among the other residents. Ironically, there were lively discussion groups at Lathrop, with people who cared about just the kind of political activism he had once taken part in, but these were not the topics he now wanted to discuss. They were not *his* discussions. He was still talking about putting together such a group when he arrived at the hospice.

Howard was not an easy presence in the Fisher Home. Even as death approached, he remained physically striking, big, imposing. In the beginning, he complained that his daughter didn't care for him and had dumped him there. He was easily irritated, anxious and demanding, and did not hesitate to let the staff know how he felt. An early assessment of him notes that he had unrealistic expectations and denied his problems. Of course, in the past, denying his problems had been a strategy that had worked amazingly well for him. According to Susan, he never really acknowledged his stroke, but kept on doing things most people would have avoided. He continued to travel to remote places, including Tibet, Nepal, and India, even to Antarctica on a Russian research vessel. In Antarctica, because he couldn't climb up and down the ladder to get off the ship, says Susan, "the Russian sailors used to just pick him up and throw him into the Zodiac— the inflatable boat—that would take them to shore, and then one of them would haul him out."

But by the end of October 2011, when he was admitted to the Fisher Home, determination and willpower were not going to be enough. Even so, he couldn't admit that he was dying. Susan remembers his early days there. "He kept saying, 'I'm not dying. I shouldn't be here.' " That was difficult for her. "I wasn't going to argue with him, but I just said, 'Well, it was the nicest place we could find.' For a long time he wouldn't acknowledge that he couldn't go back home."

Meanwhile, she and her sisters were relieved and happy with the care their father was getting, and Susan believes that Howard came to like and appreciate the place as well. Her first impression gave her a good start. "I loved the look of it—like a home. There were no indicators that it was an institution." Her twin sister, Linda Sachs, puts it even more strongly, referring to their many unhappy experiences in hospitals and nursing homes: "All the other alternatives were horrible." In the first place, she says, hospitals don't want you to die. "The dying person is in conflict with their mission. They're not set up to deal with reality. They're pretending the person is going to get better, and so not attending to the needs of the family or the person. You and your family have to fit their institutional needs and systems." By contrast, she says, for the family going through the traumas of a loved one dying, "in hospice, it's not cluttered by other experiences. It's the pure experience."

That "pure experience" was made possible because of what hospice stands for.

Howard Sachs was cared for at the Fisher Home not merely by people concerned with his physical condition, but also by staff who attended to his emotional and spiritual needs, as well as those of his family. These people, an interdisciplinary team, met every week, as they do year round, to discuss Howard's and other residents' situations, but they also kept in contact with each other between times to see that Howard and his family remained as comfortable as possible.

Susan was reassured to see that there were nurses who liked and cared about her father, and who were responsive to the need for change at various times, especially related to pain control. "That's one of the unique things about the Fisher Home. In a hospital it can take hours or even a day or two to get a medical response to a changing condition. Here, it would happen very rapidly."

When he got there, Susan was worried that he would alienate the people who would be looking after him. The caregiving job was hard, as she knew at first hand, and her father, as she also knew, could be abusive. She was happy to see that no one at the Fisher Home had "an attitude." They weren't put off by him— or if they were, they kept it to themselves. Staff were patient but firm about his demands. Huevos rancheros had to be cooked just so. Bagels were to be toasted, never heated in the microwave. People tried hard to accommodate him. Volunteers were happy to read to him even if he didn't recognize them afterward. In the case of Dr. Mark Bigda, one of the hospice's medical directors at the time, it was also a matter of being able to dish it out. Susan remembers an occasion when the doctor came in and asked Howard how he was, and her father responded that if the doctor would bend over and drop his pants, he'd show him. "And then Dr. Bigda said something to my father equally grotesque—sort of locker room stuff. It was great!" He gave as good as he got, and she could see that her father respected that.

Rabbi Benjamin Weiner, who conducted his memorial service, offered a further sense of Howard's capacity for vibrant encounters and the need to be able to roll with the punches when dealing with him. At the service, the rabbi commented on his last meeting with Howard. "As I was holding his hand and speaking with him, he suddenly opened his eyes and took a break from breathing his last to inquire of me: 'Who the fuck are *you*?' It's a question that I have often asked myself, when presuming to sit beside someone I barely know in the last stage of their life, so on one level I'm glad that he called me on it."

After weeks of being mainly hostile, Howard suddenly had a change of heart toward everybody, says Susan. "Margot Menkel, one of the aides, told me about it. One day when she walked in, he said to her, 'You look beautiful this morning.' After that he was as sweet as could be. I cried when I heard that story."

Norma Palazzo, the Fisher Home's spiritual counselor, dates that change to a moment when Howard was finally able to forgive himself for the deaths he'd caused during the war. Describing in his book the moment he'd shot a Japanese "banzai warrior" who was about to leap into his foxhole, he writes: "A strange look crossed his face, which I could see clearly. He was a young man, his eyes opened with surprise, his mouth partly open." Howard never forgot that moment. "That look on the warrior's face remains with me, 65 years later. I wish I could paint it and hang the painting and story in the United Nations as a reminder of that divine exhortation, 'Thou shalt not kill.' "

Norma was able to help him see that terrible time from a different perspective and to weigh that "unfinished business" against the good he'd done in his life. She points out, "His life was really a spiritual journey—going to the third world and serving people and trying to find that piece of humanity that connects us."

Several people who knew Howard felt they played a role in his transition to a better place emotionally. Among them was Christie Svane, a freelance editor who spent a year and a half with him, editing his writings and helping him publish his memoir. Christie saw a change in him when she gave him books about the afterlife. These books, she says, provided "medical proof that consciousness is not dependent on the brain." Since he was a neurologist, she notes, "that liberated him entirely from the fear of dying," a fear that had burdened him until then. "Before that, he expected an eternity of darkness, just nothingness."

When Howard was approaching the end—"actively dying" is the hospice term— Susan says she was surprised to find that the staff and the volunteers all wanted to go in and see him, "and I said, of course you can. Everybody can. And they would stop in the hallway and tell me little stories about what they had done with him, why they liked him. It was a revelation to me that he had had this life with them that I didn't know about, and that it was good. It was very gratifying." This woman, who had done so much to look after her father for almost two decades, felt that hospice was "the last gift I gave him."

Howard died six weeks after his admission. After keeping a vigil for several days, his daughter Nancy had returned to her home in North Carolina and Linda had gone back to New York. Susan was there in the morning, but left briefly. While she was out of the room Howard died, a few minutes after ten. "When I came back, Norma had opened the window and had covered him with a beautiful quilt, and had lit a little candle. Joan Baez, a favorite of Howard's, was playing on the CD player, and it was so peaceful and beautiful. I'll never forget it. He was peaceful. There's such a difference in the face of someone dead and someone alive, even though it's just one breath. The window was open a crack so the spirit could leave. It was kind of magical because a whole little pod of chickadees showed up at the feeder right outside his window, but then they flew away. I like to think that his spirit left in the wake of the chickadees."

Did Howard, a man who was eager to wrestle with the big questions, believe in an afterlife? "He didn't know," says Susan. "I think he hoped that there would be one. He was a scientist, so it's hard when you have a scientist's brain and attitude to believe in something that can't be replicated, shown, measured. But he became interested in that question in the later part of his life."

Susan still has the quilt that covered her father at his death. It's in a drawer. She hasn't been able to take it out yet but likes the fact that it's there. Every room in the Fisher Home has a handmade quilt on the bed. When a person dies, the quilt is given to the family.

The summer after Howard died, as a way of celebrating their joint sixtieth birthday, twins Susan and Linda Sachs came to the Fisher Home, dug up a small heart-shaped plot, and planted it with purple-flowering butterfly bushes and yellow marigolds in their father's memory.

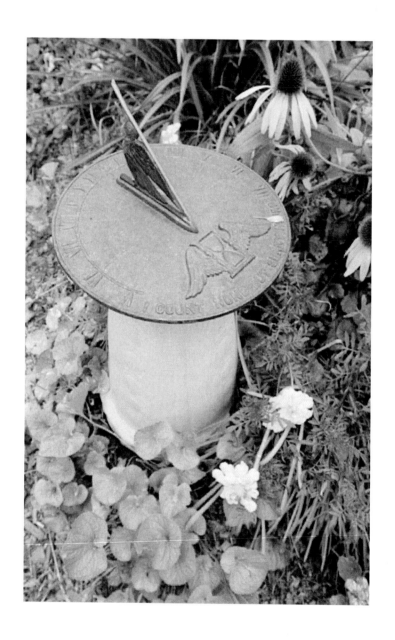

CHAPTER FOUR

Norma Palazzo:
not fear, but love

Norma Palazzo has been with the Fisher Home since the beginning. Some might call her the heart of the place, although as spiritual and bereavement counselor, she might also be said to represent its soul. If so, it is a lively, bouncy one. She's a sweet, disarming, and chatty presence, dressed stylishly in vivid colors, who loves to bake and organize celebrations. She once pulled together an outdoor wedding in two days for the daughter of a resident who could no longer travel. That's Norma's exterior, but stay with her a while and she'll surprise you with her toughness and depth, managing to connect with everyone from gruff grandfathers to sorrowing daughters, from unbending clerics of all persuasions to exasperated staff members.

One of the harder parts of her job, she says, is introducing herself as a spiritual counselor: "People tend to think it's some kind of voodoo thing." Norma's simple and complex goal is to help people who are dying identify whatever it is that has provided comfort and strength throughout their lives, to help them get back in touch with it and use it to get through the dying process. Compassion and kindness are, for her, "the only 'religion' of hospice." Those qualities can help people find love and trust, the counterweights to fear, a fear she thinks is reinforced by our society's attitudes toward death and the end of life.

Although Norma doesn't represent any religion, she also doesn't shy away from it. If a hospice resident has been active in a church or temple, she will help renew or strengthen that connection if the person wishes. She may arrange for a priest or rabbi to come and visit. At other times, she tries simply to be a compassionate presence for the resident and family at the end of life. She sometimes asks a dying person: "If you had a magic wand and you had one wish to make, what would that be? And usually they say, 'That I not die.' And then

I always say, well, that's the wish you can't have. Their second wish is usually 'To die without pain' or 'To reunite with my son who I haven't talked with in twenty years.' That's when I know what I can do to help them."

Letting go of fear is hard, she says, but she encourages people to see this time as an opportunity—like opening a window. As someone who had to overcome her own deep fear of death, she can understand how hard it is. Howard Sachs, a brave man in many ways, was angry and afraid of dying when he arrived at the hospice. He at first resisted the opportunity to come to terms with the end of his life, but with the help of Norma and others, he was able to find a kind of peace. It's a matter of trust, Norma says. "Once you can get in the door and they see that you're genuine, they let go of some of those fears."

The other part of Norma's job is as bereavement counselor, which involves keeping in touch with family members for a year after a death, offering regular support groups to those who wish it, and more informal contact and counseling to others. This is an acknowledgment of the hospice principle that the unit of care embraces the whole family and that the promise of care does not end with death.

I watch Norma at work. Very impres-
sive. She is having a conversation
with E.'s daughter N., who talks about
how difficult it all is, and is there a
chance that a physical therapist might
be able to bring her mother back, yet
knowing that really there isn't. She
describes a conversation she's had
with her mother about heaven, and how
they'd meet up there and Mom could
keep house for them all again. Norma
is good at listening and trying to
move N. in the direction of coming to
terms with this imminent death. Yes,
it will be a shock, even if you've
been expecting it.

**

W. is relatively new here. I haven't
seen him until today because I thought
he didn't want to be visited. His door
is kept closed. He's fifty-eight and
dying of pancreatic cancer. He also
had polio as a kid, which has now
recurred in that cruel postpolio syndrome, which mimics the symptoms of
the original disease. Things pretty
quiet today, so I thought I'd give him
a try. I say hello, tell him my name,
and shake his hand. OK if I stay for a
few minutes? Sure, he says, and we

wind up talking for half an hour. He's
a rugged-looking guy's guy who likes
to hunt with his buddies. A list of
his favorite foods posted on the
fridge includes mostly meat and pota-
toes. Breakfast is five scrambled eggs
and bacon. He doesn't eat at the table
with others, only in his room.

He grew up in one of those little
towns on Route 2A, he tells me.
Worked last in Gardner in an office
job, but before that in construction--
lots of big machines, also as a
mechanic, as a manager of liquor
stores and restaurants. Went out to
Colorado at one point, when the woman
he was with went there, but couldn't
find real work. His sister is out
there. Likes her, but there's a
brother he doesn't. Brother is a real
strict Catholic, the way they were
all brought up, though W. isn't anymore. He got mad at his brother, who
inherited their parents' house and
then complained he hadn't gotten any
money. W. thinks that when the
brother goes to confession, the
priest would have to bring his lunch
and dinner while the brother con-
fesses all his terrible sins. Must
take all day.

Likes the Fisher Home, hated the
place he was in before, a nursing home
where he shared a room with a guy who
didn't know who or where he was. The
director had promised that they were
moving him in there temporarily, but
that wasn't the case. "She lied to me,
and I told her I don't let people lie
to me. When the doctor came to tell me
about my cancer, I told him, give it
to me straight. I don't want anyone
lying to me." He plans to have his
ashes mixed with those of his late
dog--picture in a frame by the bed-
side--and scattered in the Colorado
mountains.

He's selling his house, so only
brought a few things with him--his
wheelchair (he was already wheelchair-
bound), his shower chair, and a few
other things. He wouldn't be needing
the rest. He hasn't wanted to talk
much with volunteers so far. I got
lucky. I learn that he collects
antique cars. A topic for our next
conversation?

W.'s stance about lying makes me
think of a passage in Tolstoy's
wrenching story "The Death of Ivan
Ilych":

What tormented Ivan Ilych most was the deception, the lie, which for some reason they all accepted, that he was not dying but was simply ill, and that he only need keep quiet and undergo a treatment and then something very good would result. He however knew that do what they would nothing would come of it, only still more agonizing suffering and death. This deception tortured him—their not wishing to admit what they all knew and what he knew, but wanting to lie to him concerning his terrible condition, and wishing and forcing him to participate in that lie. Those lies—lies enacted over him on the eve of his death and destined to degrade this awful, solemn act to the level of their visitings, their curtains, their sturgeon for dinner— were a terrible agony for Ivan Ilych.*

---

* Leo Tolstoy, "The Death of Ivan Ilych," in *Ivan Ilych, Hadji Murad and Other Stories* (London: Oxford University Press, 1957), 50.

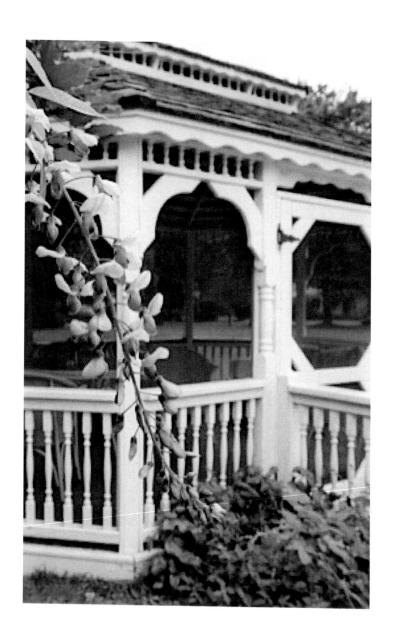

CHAPTER FIVE

KATHY CURTIS:
THE HIGHEST STANDARDS

ATHY CURTIS, AUBURN-HAIRED, impeccably turned out, seems taller than she is because of her elegant bearing. She is always responsive to a question from staff, volunteers, or family members, but she's not looking for someone to talk to, does not hang out in the hallways or kitchen chatting. You'll find her in her office. She is here to work, and hers is a big job. It is, in her words, "to make sure clinical excellence prevails in all areas." These are matters of life and death, not to mention continued accreditation and licensing for the Fisher Home. As clinical director, she oversees the day-to-day activities of all of the clinical staff—nurses and aides. She is the one who sees to it that the i's are dotted and the t's crossed on the mountains of state and federally required documents. In addition to the weekly inter-disciplinary meeting of clinical and managerial staff, she holds a clinical staff meeting every month. There, nurses and aides go over anything that's happened in the house, "anything that's good, that's bad, that needs to change," she says.

Kathy is also responsible for much of the contact with insurance companies, updating them on the patients' care plans. When bills come in, she looks at them to make sure they're correct in terms of any-thing clinical.

Nursing was what she always knew she wanted to do, although it was a goal that had to be suspended during the first years of her marriage. After completing her R.N., she worked in an oncology unit in a Boston hospital. That was a defining experience for her, she says: "I saw too much suffering that I felt didn't need to happen. People were being treated—futilely treated—

right up to the end, when they maybe could have had some good, quality time with their families. The doctors were always pushing for the next treatment, for the next experimental drug. And that just left a bad taste in my mouth." By the time she left there after a couple of years, she had decided she wanted to go into hospice work. A job opened up in Worcester, and from then on, she says, "It was just a passion. I can't imagine doing any other kind of nursing."

Day to day, Kathy is responsible for seeing that patients are receiving the right medications, that pain is being controlled, that other symptoms are being managed. She is on call, and nurses can reach her whatever the hour. If, as sometimes happens, she can't answer a question or make a decision on her own, she'll call on the medical director. She does all the hiring of nursing staff—advertising, interviewing, and making the final employment decisions. Meanwhile, she's also formulating policies and procedures for how the staff functions. For instance, she has increased the amount of time a new nurse spends in orientation, working on the floor with a mentor. The reason for that change, she points out, is that hospice is special. "You can have a wonderful nurse who just hasn't had hospice experience, and they need to see all of the different areas and know what to do in a crisis situation." Like doctors' training, nurses' education is typically aimed at a cure. Hospice is not about curing, but rather about comfort, choice, and dignity at the end of life.

Kathy is also involved in community education. She and director Maxine Stein have been going out to medical centers, senior centers, and other community venues to let people know more about the Fisher Home, especially to let them know that care is also available in people's homes. That is, in fact, the organization's mission, says Kathy—to serve the community. Often a group will invite her to come and speak about what hospice is. "There's still confusion about this even among doctors, so some of it is about trying to inform them as well." It's important, too, she says, to educate staff in doctors' offices, since they are often the "gate-keepers," helping to make recommendations and referrals about care for patients.

When families come in, she usually sits down with them to explain everything they need to know— "especially the things that we normally *won't* do, like IV fluids when people can't swallow anymore." Standard hospice procedure in this regard is based on the understanding that as a person dies and bodily systems shut down, the cells are less able to handle nutrition or fluids. For that reason, pushing food or liquids only increases the dying person's discomfort. For most people not familiar with this principle, it is hard to relinquish the impulse to feed and hydrate a loved one. But a dying person can be kept comfortable with mouth swabs and sips of water. In very rare cases— only a couple of times since the hospice opened—they have given IV fluids to someone whose thirst was a source of discomfort, says Kathy.

She will also explain to families their rights. "The first thing I do is give them the state Department of Public Health hotline number, and I let them know that if there are ever any issues or problems, they need to let us know first and we will try to take care of those issues. And if they feel the problem hasn't been solved, they can call the DPH hotline, and they will investigate." Early in the Fisher Home's history there was one such investigation, and the department came but found nothing wrong. "It's important for people to know that they have another place to go, other than us," says Kathy.

She also explains the patient's responsibilities.

To whatever extent possible, the dying person needs to let hospice staff know what he or she is experiencing, "to let us know if you're having more pain, if there's a symptom that you're experiencing so that we can do something to help you." The patient who is still conscious needs to know all these things. For those no longer able to speak, the staff, who are always updating their skills, are well attuned to nonverbal signals of distress and can respond to those.

If Norma represents the hospice's soul, Kathy Curtis is surely its backbone. Without her strength, expertise, and reliability, the place would not function. For a time, between Greg Keochakian's departure and Maxine Stein's arrival, Kathy worked two jobs, as clinical director and executive director. For over a year, she not only had to deal with the medical side of the organization, but also its finances and human resources, along with the day-to-day physical problems of the building and its grounds. Now that Maxine is in charge of the physical plant and all things financial, and accountant Donna Sarro handles human resources, Kathy is delighted to turn all her attention to caring for dying people, a full-time job in itself, and one she loves.

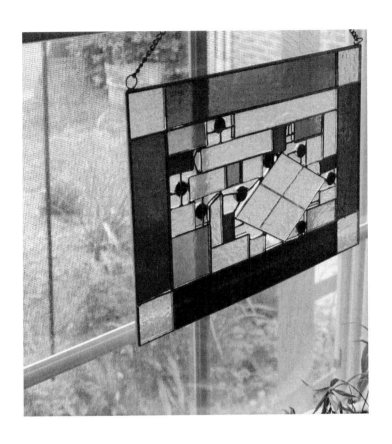

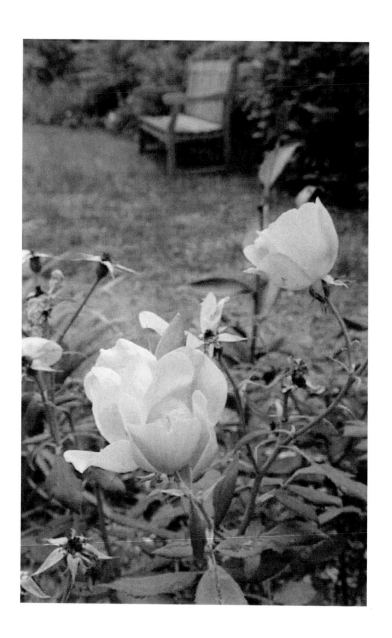

CHAPTER SIX

INTERDISCIPLINARY TEAM MEETING: REVISITING THE WEEK

NORMA OPENS THE MEETING by tapping a wooden mallet on a Tibetan singing bowl, a gentle but penetrating sound. There is silence, then she reads a poem by Mary Oliver, from a collection titled *Thirst*.

THE USES OF SORROW

(In my sleep I dreamed this poem)

Someone I loved once gave me
A box full of darkness.

It took me years to understand
that this, too, was a gift.

The readings that open these interdisciplinary team meetings always have a spiritual message, usually a positive or enlightening one. They tend to be multi-cultural and not overtly religious, although, Norma says, "I mix them up, sometimes find things that are specific to holidays." There are a few quiet comments about the poem's wisdom before the group gets down to its weekly business.

The Fisher Home team meets every week for an hour or more. These meetings embody a way of doing things that is central to hospice—people from different disciplines regularly exchanging information, observations, and views about each patient. Although this kind of exchange goes on all the time in patients' rooms, in hallways, in offices, the weekly meeting is the time to formalize and record everyone's observations and concerns, to make sure everyone knows what the others know. It is also a time to update each patient's plan of care, both for the patient and for family members. Staff may suggest a family meeting with the social worker and nurse to explain any changes in that plan.

Houseplants flourish on the conference room's windowsills. In addition to Norma, the group includes medical director Dr. Paul Berman, clinical director Kathy Curtis, social worker Priscilla White, volunteer coordinator Ilsa Myers, CNA team leader Jenn Messinger, nurse Matt DeLuca, and community nurse Maria Rivera.

Volunteers may come to the meeting, and families of patients are always invited to take part and discuss their concerns.

First the deaths. Ilsa reads off the names, and Matt, the nurse in charge of summarizing this week's notes from different nurses and aides, describes the final hours of those who died—who was there, how it went, how the families seem to be coping. Others add their observations and concerns. In the case of one woman who died, the family at first thought she was too heavily sedated, but then realized how much pain she was in and how near she was to death, so came to understand that the medication was appropriate. The family had been there all the last day. After they left to go out for dinner, the woman died. This is not an unusual occurrence, say experienced hospice staff. Some people seem to prefer to die without family around. It is seen as a choice.

Priscilla observes that one of the woman's sons will have the hardest time. Norma takes note of this, since in her role as bereavement counselor she will contact the family, provide them with written materials, and begin her regular schedule of keeping in touch for the year to come, at whatever level they seem to need.

Next, Matt reports on new patients. One woman, ninety-five, has an arterial occlusion in one leg, which is blue, cold, and swollen. She comes with a further diagnosis of debility and dementia. She has spent eight years in a nursing home and came here from a local hospital's intensive care unit. She has Do Not Resuscitate and Do Not Intubate orders, but in the hospital she was getting no pain medication. Dr. Berman is appalled at what he sees as neglect. "This is unbelievable," he says, and explains that even though the patient was not alert or able to communicate, the hospital staff should have known that this is an incredibly painful condition. The woman is now getting the proper pain relief. Her daughter has brought her prescription of the narcotic Roxanol from the hospital to the hospice. And, says Matt, she has also brought ice cream. There are smiles around the table. This is typical hospice care—sophisticated attention to alleviating pain while also providing the simple and basic pleasures of life, including comfort food.

Another person admitted in the past few days is a ninety-three-year-old man who has clearly said he wants to die. He has been an active member of his retirement community up until a few weeks ago, when he suddenly became depleted. Doctors found an abdominal mass and biopsied it, but he didn't want the results, doesn't want treatment, wants to go fast. The family was having a hard time, but seemed also to be coping with his last days. Dr. Berman says that if there had been a diagnosis, it might be lymphoma, which is treatable. (In fact the patient died the next day.) The family was feeling the end of things in a lot of ways—the death of an uncle a few weeks earlier, the sale of the last parcel of family land. But, reports Norma, "They seem to be in pretty good agreement about dealing with his last days—and they love this place." This is important, since families are seen as part of the unit of care in hospice. But there are practical reasons, too. The Fisher Home depends on its good reputation to bring in more residents. And beyond that, there are potential legal issues—an unhappy family is more likely to sue, something that has never happened here.

Another patient, an eighty-five-year-old woman, is dying of cancer of the bladder, ovaries, and vagina. Matt lists her many medications, given through patches or a CADD (computerized ambulatory drug delivery) pump, an efficient method for administering morphine. This is not an intravenous device, but rather delivers medication subcutaneously, under the skin. Intravenous devices are rarely used at the Fisher Home, usually only when a patient arrives with one in place. Hospice policy is to be as physically unintrusive as possible. This resident is not eating, and drinking only sips. Norma reports that the woman's family has some concern that she's overmedicated, and her husband complained that she's sleeping all the time. He made this comment to Norma in his wife's room, whereupon the patient—a retired nurse—spoke up quite clearly: "What else am I supposed to do?" The husband, says Norma, is "the cutest ninety-five-year-old, still cutting wood for his neighbors." She thinks he feels quite at home here.

Another resident is described as "quite manic" lately. This is evidently characteristic of the type of dementia she suffers from, which is known as Lewy body disease, the second most common type of dementia after Alzheimer's. A darkened room, soft music, gentle touch, and quiet company can help, with also the possibility of an extra dose of an antipsychotic medication.

Recertification is an issue for several residents. This is always difficult, since people usually come to the hospice in very bad shape but after a time may improve, meaning that they have to "graduate" to a nursing home or assisted living facility. One of the things that typically happens when a person arrives at the Fisher Home is that medications, except for those used for symptom control, are gradually eliminated. And since the side effects of multiple medications often make people sicker, the resident may get his appetite back, may start to be more mobile, more communicative and alert. The care, it might be said, is too good, and the person who is no longer in decline can no longer be considered a hospice patient, which means that most insurance policies will not pay for care. This is the situation with two of the residents this week. There is some discussion about how the first man's status can be assessed. He has been recertified for another sixty-day period, but after that, what? Is he losing weight? This would indicate decline. Kathy Curtis, the clinical director, says there's a problem with weighing him. They can't put him into the Hoyer lift because he's so rigid. Ilsa asks, couldn't we assess his weight by measuring his midarm circumference? Dr. Berman points out that anyone with dementia will be in decline, but that may not be enough for Medicare's rules about recertification.

The other resident, Dr. Gerard Sterling, has a slow-acting brain tumor, is bed-bound, partly blind, and has little recent memory. Unfortunately, he is also quite aware of his situation and is intensely anxious about the prospect of having to leave the Fisher Home. He has been here before, had to leave when his condition plateaued, and then returned after he declined again. It's possible, someone suggests, that if Medicare won't pay for him to stay, his catastrophic insurance might cover him here. Various insurance possibilities are discussed, and Priscilla asks whether he could stay here as a private-pay hospice patient, then spend down and go over to Medicaid. All of these options will be looked into.

Matt reports that another patient with widespread cancer is definitely declining, sleeping more, experiencing more nausea and pain. He lists a number of medications they're using to try to control her symptoms. Until recently, she has been cheerful and talkative, but now she doesn't want to be visited by volunteers, wants to see only her partner, who is trying to keep her occupied, taking her outside, playing games. She feels better when she talks, but forgets everything pretty quickly. Another nurse suggests that her medications may be making her sick. Dr. Berman says: Let's take away all the meds except for treating the nausea. Kathy says a subcutaneous pump might help with the nausea, but also wonders whether the patient still has enough body fat to hold the pump. Maybe on her thigh, she suggests.

One other patient has been here for "respite," allowing his wife time to get some rest and think about what happens next. He is a big man with Parkinson's disease and some dementia, but although he needs a lot of help moving safely, his wife really wants him at home. Kathy says he has a low Karnofsky Performance Status Score, a classification of functional impairment, indicating that he cannot take care of many daily activities. She says the family was on board for him to be here when they last talked, but if he stays as long as six months, they will need a long-term-care plan. As a veteran, he is eligible for residence in the Holyoke Soldiers Home, a well-respected long-term-care facility about fifteen miles away.

The longest discussion of the day has to do with a patient who has been discharged from hospice care but has remained at the Fisher Home because her family can't find a suitable alternative. A feisty, independent-spirited woman with advanced Parkinson's, she had refused to call for help when she needed to get up, and a few days ago fell and now likely has a nondisplaced hip fracture. She's in a lot of pain, is very difficult for staff to move, and isn't eating. The first doctor who examined her said she should be discharged to a hospital where they could pin the hip, but the family has said they don't want surgery. What is the Fisher Home's responsibility here? Jenn asks if we might have access to a mobile X-ray machine to see what has actually happened. Dr. Berman, agreeing with the first doctor, says she should go to the hospital, otherwise she could "throw an embolus," a life-threatening blood clot. Furthermore, the broken bone can come through the skin, and then no matter how much morphine you give her, it won't help and she'll go to the hospital in agony. There are legal issues here in addition to all the medical and humanitarian ones—could we be considered neglectful? Kathy says: If the family doesn't respond, we might have to call Protective Services, a state agency that deals with elder abuse. We can't take care of her because she's no longer a hospice patient. Finally Dr. Berman says: The family has to take responsibility. Call them. That is what they will do.

The meeting adjourns with some cheerful banter about the breast pump Maria will be using when the room clears out. She's storing milk for her six-month-old in the house refrigerator.

A source of amusement for the living
room crowd is my weekly cleaning of
the fish tank. This involves putting my
arm deep into the tank and rooting
around with the siphon to remove the
old water, then bringing in buckets of
clean water from the laundry room to
replace it. The fish don't seem to
mind, and M., among others, finds it
quite entertaining.

An aide and a nurse are talking
about their "favorite" patients. The
nurse prefers people who want to know
about their illness--who want to talk,
ask questions--since she likes teaching people. The aide feels differently,
preferring the strong, silent types.
This is an attitude I've encountered
with another aide who expressed frus-
tration with a highly articulate woman
who wanted to talk through every stage
of her dying. "I can't stand it," said
the aide. "She wants to process everything!"

***

Things are quiet at the hospice, so I
bring my gardening clothes and tools,
and wind up pruning the enormous

rhododendrons obscuring the front and
side windows. A satisfying, sweaty
task. I manage to take a piece out of
my finger with my own pruners. Luckily
there are nurses and plenty of Band-
Aids.

E. is still here. I chat with her
daughter. The staff thinks the family
is "in denial" about E., who barely
speaks anymore, although family members describe conversations with her.
They like to have her nicely dressed
(beautiful nightgowns, including one
white cotton with heavy lace embroi-
dery over her gaunt collarbones),
fingernails painted. Her head is pretty
much a skull. I would guess she's in
her last phase.

I "meet" S., a new person who is
unresponsive. When a friend of hers
comes in I leave, then learn a few
minutes later that S. has died.

***

A new patient, T., late-stage pancreatic cancer, in terrible pain. Staff
very stretched when I arrive, so I do
some cooking for the next meal after
finding enough vegetables for a (frozen)

shrimp stir-fry. Several residents--
including J., who is here for a
respite stay--need to have their food
ground up, but nurse Lucy Fandel has
suggested that I cook something for
residents Isabel Glass and Lee Shotland, both of whom, she says, "like to
be able to tell what they're eating."

Meanwhile, many of T.'s relatives
are here for lunch, and for the day.
On the fridge is an enormous list of
the foods he likes--quite poignant,
since he has been vomiting steadily.
I get his teenage son to help with
refilling the fish tank after I clean
it. Ilsa thanks me for "normalizing"
things for him.

                    ***

Ilsa has called to say that someone
I know is now at the Fisher Home: Sara
Wolff. Though not a close friend, I
have known Sara for decades and we
have remained friendly. Her children
and ours were in school together, and
we were both involved in early phases
of the women's movement in the late
1960s. A few months ago I had encountered her husband, Michael, in a local

bookstore, and he'd told me she was
ill with some sort of blood disease
and was in a nursing home. I'm wondering how to greet her. Hi, Sara, good
to see you. Hi, Sara, sorry you're
ill. Hi, Sara, I'm glad you're here.
This is the first time someone
I know well who is also alert has
arrived here.

When I stop in to see Sara, she
solves my problem by greeting me first,
then showing me the card she's sending
to friends telling them what has been
happening to her. The card has a lovely
color photo of the clematis from her
garden, and the text is simple and
declarative: I have a blood disease;
I am now in the Fisher Home; please
write to me rather than calling or
visiting. She is absolutely clear. One
of the aides has asked her about her
spirituality, and she had to say she
was afraid she didn't have any. On
second thought, maybe it has to do
with her garden. I say maybe those of
us who think of ourselves as humanists
are harder to pin down in that respect.
She is avoiding one staff member,
whose "perkiness" irritates her--"She

perked in here the other day." Sara
still has a good sharp edge.

She's had a haircut, she says with
a wide smile. Cheryl Poulin, one of
the aides, cut it for her. This is a
wonderful place in other ways, too,
she says. "You get anything you want
to eat."

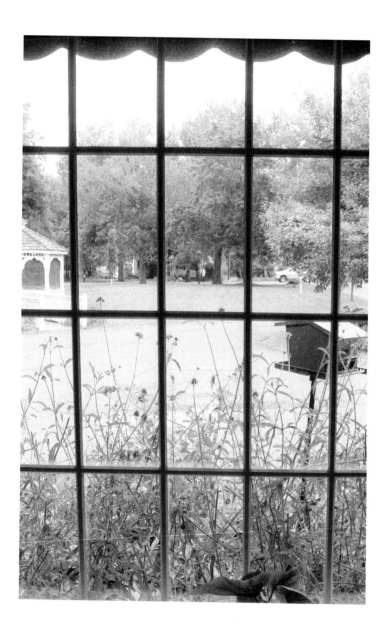

CHAPTER SEVEN

SARA WOLFF:
MAKING HER OWN DECISIONS

SARA WOLFF'S STORY couldn't be more different from Howard Sachs'. Howard came to the Fisher Home struggling to deny the fact that he was dying. By contrast, in July 2011, when Sara understood that her illness was fatal, that the current treatment was not helping but only making her more uncomfortable, she took matters into her own hands and decided to come to the Fisher Home. No less determined or courageous in her own way than Howard, she had led a full life of work and family. A psychotherapist who had retired as director of mental health at Amherst Medical Associates, she was the mother of three and grandmother of six. Unlike Howard, who had a New York slum childhood, she was born into a comfortable upper-middle-class existence in Nashville,

Tennessee, where her businessman father, Milton Starr, had been affiliated with the southern writers' group known as the Fugitives and had worked in the Roosevelt administration during World War II. Unlike Howard, who put himself through college on the G.I. Bill, Sara's family was able to send her to Sarah Lawrence, a private women's college.

Like Howard, when she arrived at the Fisher Home, she had recently self-published a book; but this one, which came out in 2010, was not her own story, though she was deeply involved in it. *Vital Aging* was the product of conversations she had generated with a group of older women in Amherst over the course of seven years. It chronicles their thoughts about such topics as living arrangements for the elderly, health problems and health care, and how to face the end of life. Ironically, it was just the sort of group that Howard Sachs might have wanted to be part of.

Sara radiated an intense calm. Her illness began with acute back pain, which led to the discovery of a blood disorder, myelodysplastic syndrome, a preleukemic condition that can be mild or severe. Sara's was severe. After several months in hospitals and nursing homes for treatment with chemotherapy and blood transfusions, and after acquiring a debilitating intestinal infection known as *Clostridium difficile*, she returned home for a while, with help from the local visiting nurses association. Eventually she decided not to endure further treatments, which were only making her more miserable, and to give up the struggle to make complicated home-care arrangements.

Sara already knew more than most people did about the Fisher Home, since she had been part of the Friends of Hospice, the group that had originally worked to open such a residence. She had followed the hospice's development with great interest. One chapter of her book begins with the following observation about the Vital Aging group she had led: "There was a matter-of-fact tone in the way people spoke about death. And we frequently quoted Lynn [one of the group's members]: 'You can't get out of this life alive.' " This down-to-earth and slightly humorous-ironic tone is the one Sara herself could be depended upon to use. It was easy to talk with her about final things and her thoughts about them. She knew that some of her friends were surprised that she had decided to die someplace other than her beautiful Amherst home, surrounded by books and objects chosen over a lifetime, next to the garden she loved so much. She was clear-eyed about this. She did not want to have to think about possessions or responsibilities, except for the ones she had chosen for this room in which she now lived. Though Sara was quite secular in her beliefs, the room felt a lot like a pilgrim's cell, a sacred space. She did not watch TV or listen to music, and did not encourage much company. Her computer was banned. It was a space where her husband, Michael, her children, grandchildren, and a short list of friends could come and visit. She encouraged others to write to her, since she was sleeping a lot and lacked the energy to deal with the many acquaintances who wanted to call or stop by. Besides, as a woman of considerable beauty and some vanity, she hated the way she now looked. She had lost a great deal of weight and the ravages of her disease were showing on her skin. At the end, Michael said, he came to understand what the phrase "skin and bones" really meant.

Michael and Sara had had a marriage that he describes as "a continual romance." The June after her death, he noted, was the fifty-eighth anniversary of their meeting. That was a Saturday, and he had proposed on the following Wednesday. She went with him to Indiana University, where he had a job teaching English, and in 1970 to Amherst, where he taught at the University of Massachusetts, specializing in Victorian studies, until his retirement in 1992. Michael describes himself as a "militant atheist," and although Sara shared his secular outlook, unlike him "she didn't share it in the aggressive way." He's convinced that she did not backslide from her secular views, and continues to be amazed at "how strong she was, and unafraid." Michael doesn't believe in another life, but he does believe in memory, and sees his marriage and the loss of Sara as "the most important of my memories." He quotes Ludwig Wittgenstein, who said that death is not an event in life. Michael finds this formulation helpful.

When she arrived at the Fisher Home, Sara sent out the cards she had showed me to her entire mailing list with the message informing her friends that she was there, and that they should write rather than phone or show up. Later, when a kind friend brought a hummingbird feeder and a pot of red salvia to attract finches to her window, she was grateful but expressed mixed feelings. She had gotten used to looking out that window, watching the clouds roll over an austere view—the hospice's roofline with its air-conditioning vents. Now there was more visual complication there, something to pull her attention away from the inner order she was trying to make.

She made maximum use of her time at the Fisher Home, enjoying the food up until the end, especially the elaborate breakfasts made on weekends by volunteer George Maston. She was thinking ahead: She and Michael had already bought their burial plots, but she now wanted to consult with people about planning a memorial service. She kept a journal of her final days, small spiral-bound notebooks with blue covers that she wrote in by hand. She was doing what she had done as a psychologist, recording observations about someone's life, but this time the life she was observing was her own.

Among other things, she pondered the question of how you make a case for hospice without saying you're "giving up." The rhetoric around disease is so combative—people battle cancer; they're survivors, winners. For many, including doctors, not treating a disease feels like losing. Friends suggested that she seemed to be working on another project, called *Vital Dying*.

She saw a lot of her children, who came up from New York on the weekends; and two of her granddaughters spent the summer in a friend's nearby condo, visiting, helping out with practical matters, keeping people's spirits up. Sometimes Michael sat by her bed and read aloud from classic works of English literature—*Pride and Prejudice*, among others.

At Collective Copies in Amherst, whose Levellers Press had published Sara's book, a discreet note was attached to the copy on display there. It read:

> Sara Wolff, Levellers author, has requested that her share from the sale of her book, *Vital Aging*, go to the Fisher Home. She has been diagnosed with MDS, a rare and serious blood disorder, and despite treatment and good care, her health has continued to decline, and she has decided she is ready for hospice.

She may have been ready, but her family was not, especially her three children. It took them a while to understand and agree with her decision. But Sara was also anticipating their difficulties, the difficulties of many people when they think about hospice. Says her daughter Judith, "Her choice to go into hospice—she was worried that we thought she was giving up." Sara asked Michael and Judith to go and look at the Fisher

Home. At this point Judith became more involved, in effect the designated offspring. Their first visit didn't produce much of an impression, except that the hospice was smaller, a little more homey than the places Sara had already been. Only a week before, they had been in the local emergency room getting Sara a blood transfusion. "So it felt like a big deal when she was talking about going to hospice and refusing any more medical treatment," says Judith. "But it was also clear how uncomfortable and how awful all the treatments were."

One of Sara's friends called Judith and said, "Your mom really wants to move to the hospice. She wants you guys to be there for her when she moves, and she's having a hard time conveying how much she wants to go." At this point, a room became available, and Sara's oncologist certified that Sara was hospice-appropriate. So Judith, her father, her daughter, and her daughter's boyfriend moved her. Judith remembers that it all seemed "incredibly unceremonious." Still, she says, "I'm sure it's never what you expect. As prepared as my mother was—I don't know anybody who could have been more prepared, and also in control—I don't have any notion that this was not the scariest and most awful, terrible thing for her to go through. But the fact that she was in control was incredibly important for her. For her kids, she would never say how afraid she was, but I'm hoping that she had people at the hospice— and her friends."

In mid-September, two months into her stay at the hospice, Sara complained of being bored, irritated by everything, including the blue sky. This was all taking longer than she had expected, and the doctors couldn't give her a good prediction for how much longer it would be. She was not in pain, but very tired. She couldn't read much. She thought about bringing in her laptop to write on, but then she would have to contend with everything that was on it—delete old files, look at e-mails. Her children suggested getting her a new computer so that she could start fresh, but she wasn't sure about that. In the end, a computer never entered the room.

Sara was pleased with the way the Fisher Home had been the catalyst for bringing her family together. She didn't mean that they had been kept apart by con-flict or disagreements, but that it gave them a place to come and be with each other without having to take care of her. Indeed the hospice was fulfilling one of its major goals, the chance for family members to resume their roles as spouses, children, and grandchildren, without the extra burden of caregiving.

One day in late summer, one of Sara's granddaughters arranged for a tabla player to come and perform in the house's living room. A young Indian man sat on the floor and played this traditional set of variously tuned drums while Violet, the granddaughter, who had spent time in India, danced. For this Sara made a rare foray out of her room, and her family and a few friends were invited.

In early November, Sara began to weaken and the signs of her disease were more visible in the dark bruiselike lesions—called ecchymoses—that appeared under her skin. Sara had appreciated the directness of Dr. Berman, whom Judith describes as a "tell-it-like-it-is guy." He had told Sara that she would just get weaker, not have pain. A few days before her death, Berman told Michael that Sara had had a bleed to her brain, most likely the beginning of the end. On November 11, the nurse on duty called her family to say that that end was near. She died that day, with family members at her side.

Sometimes it's the little things that keep coming up after a death. Judith thinks about a snafu with Sara's hearing aids. They were taken to be repaired, but the technician wasn't on duty, so there was a delay of several days in getting them back to Sara. Judith keeps a notepad from the Fisher Home where staff were writing things down because Sara couldn't hear. Says Judith, "Every time I see that now, it makes me sad that it was really hard for her to communicate at the last."

On December 15, 2012, three days before Sara and Michael's fifty-seventh wedding anniversary, several hundred people assembled in the Jewish Community of Amherst's large, well-lit space to acknowledge Sara's life and mourn her absence. Both Sara and Michael were ethnically Jewish, but the location was the only nod to that fact. The event was reverent and loving, but in no way religious. Family members, friends, and colleagues spoke; poems written at various times by Michael to Sara were read; the grandchildren sang "Tomorrow"; letters she received in the hospice were read aloud; and there was a sing-along to a couple of Sara's favorites: "The Riddle" ("I gave my love a cherry") and "Don't Fence Me In." Finally, Michael rose to speak, something he had not exactly planned. He said that he didn't want to sound "spiritual" but that he felt Sara was still with him, and always would be.

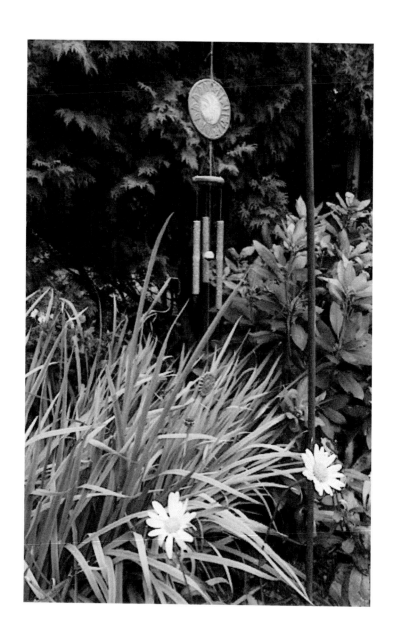

CHAPTER EIGHT

LUCY FANDEL:
COMPASSION PLUS SKILL

EVERYONE WHO HAS SPENT ANY TIME at the Fisher Home remembers Lucy Fandel, a sturdy, white-haired woman who never seems to sit down. Lucy greets everyone like a respected friend, a warmth she combines with an intense seriousness about her profession. "Since I was a child," she says, "I wanted to be a nurse." But life took her elsewhere, and after teaching high school science in Guatemala and running an educational enterprise in Africa, she returned to the States to teach adult literacy in Boston, Springfield, and Holyoke. Only then did she go to nursing school, completing her R.N. when she was sixty-four. Her background has always been in the teaching of adults, something she sees as an important aspect of nursing.

She had been good friends with Barbara Snoek, whom she'd known from the Northampton Society of Friends. Lucy was still in nursing school when the hospice opened up, and Barbara said, "I want you there when you get your nursing degree." Lucy applied and was hired.

Her routine at the hospice is like that of the other nurses. She gets there early for her 8 a.m. to 4 p.m. shift—by 7 or 7:30—so that if there are new residents, she can learn about them before she takes over. She then gets the night nurse's report. Together, they tally the narcotics, making sure none are unaccounted for, after which Lucy hits the ground running, checking in with each patient and giving people their morning medications. Later she'll go back again, spending a bit more time finding out whether they're comfortable, what their needs are. "It might be just a cup of tea or it might be pain medicine. Curtains open or shut? Do they want to sleep some more or get washed up?"

She tries to coordinate her visits with the aide on

duty, so that when the aide goes in to change an incontinence brief, for instance, Lucy can check the condition of that patient's skin, if that has been a concern. "An awful lot is asked of the aides at the Fisher Home," Lucy explains. "It's a balancing act to have the patients' needs and desires primary and still get their other work done," such as laundry and cooking.

As all the nurses do, Lucy takes notes all day long, and at the end of the shift, referring to these observations, she gives her report orally to the next nurse. Then she'll write up the notes more formally to document her shift. If there's an admission, there's interviewing and even more paperwork. Each patient is assigned a primary nurse, and once a week that nurse fills out a head-to-toe assessment known as a "home visit," a six-page form that documents every phase of the resident's current condition.

Lucy is keenly aware that aside from the comfort and freedom from pain a hospice offers, different people want and need different things at the end of their lives. Some want company and stimulating conversation; some want silence and solitude; some want music or TV. You can learn about these preferences in snippets of conversation with the resident or the family, she says—all she really has time for as she makes her rounds. But she also sees that it's important for caregivers to share something of themselves as well, to find someplace they can connect. She's found a bond with several residents because she's lived in different parts of the world and can talk with them about it. "It's all about comfort," says Lucy, "and being known for who they are, respected for who they are, having that recognized."

As a "new nurse," Lucy knows that there's much to be learned about death and dying. She considers herself a spiritual person, though not a religious one. Like many of the hospice staff, she believes in an afterlife, though she doesn't know what it's like: "My beliefs are kind of eclectic." The people she lived with in Africa believed that we're all one community, "the child in the womb not yet born, those of us we can see, and those that have gone before." That makes sense to her, she says. She tries to keep reading, tries to grow "so that I can minister to people in ways that aren't just drugs."

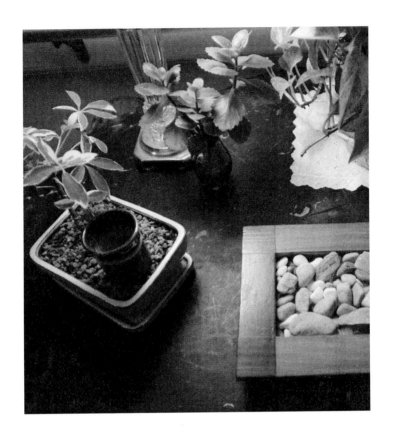

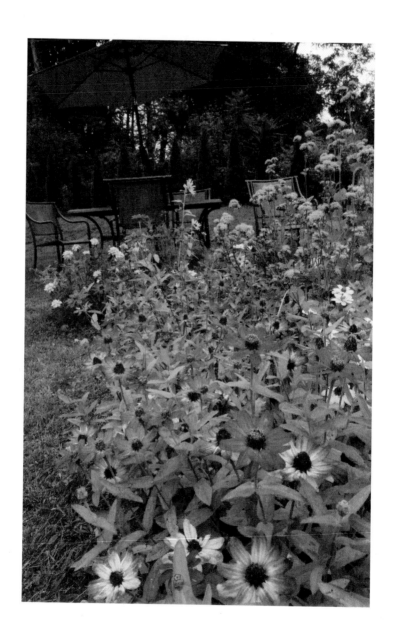

CHAPTER NINE

DOCUMENTATION:
FOR THE RECORD

A T A CONFERENCE SPONSORED by the National Hospice and Palliative Care Organization in 2011, the keynote speaker was Valerie Maasdorp, director of a hospice in Zimbabwe. Her witty and wise talk on the need for resilience in hospice work sent her audience away realizing how lucky they were to live in a first-world country not ravaged by AIDS, by political instability, or by insecure or nonexistent basic services—electricity, roads, medical supplies. In Zimbabwe, she said, you never expect things to work. She described her morning dash out of bed to get her water boiling for tea before the utilities shut off for the next few hours.

She painted a sometimes grim picture, yet she painted it with grit and good humor that exemplified the resilience she was advocating. When she told them what she did, people at cocktail parties would respond: "You must be mad or incredibly tough, or else a tender-hearted do-gooder!" No, she would say, "I am privileged. What I do feeds my soul. There is vibrancy, friendship. It is demanding and daunting, but also energizing. As a hospice worker, if you step over the line to feel pain, it costs you. But we need to do that, to walk beside our clients. Then we can make a difference, and not everyone can say that."

During the previous day's conference sessions, she had been impressed with how much talk there was about documentation, something she doesn't have to bother with. "We don't get any money, so we don't need documentation," she explained, to general laughter.

In the United States as in Zimbabwe, hospice workers walk beside their clients, but here they must record every footstep. Documentation is key to staying licensed, and to staying afloat financially. At the Fisher Home all nurses and aides keep clear, chronological notes about the condition and care of patients. Volunteers, too, keep track of their comings and goings, and are asked to write narrative notes at the end of each visit about residents they've spent time with. All licensed hospices must complete massive amounts of documentation, a full array of paperwork for each person who enters their care. A yard-wide file drawer in Kathy Curtis' office contains multiple blank copies of the dozens of forms that must accompany all admissions and the course of every patient's stay until death and the body's removal from the hospice. This documentation is required by the state and federal agencies—Medicare, Medicaid, Mass Health—that license the hospice and pay for treatment.

Kept in each patient's chart are also optional documents that the person may arrive with, add to, or change during their stay: powers of attorney, health care proxies, and a new document seen as an improvement over the older Do Not Resuscitate orders. This is a series of decisions known as MOLST (Medical Orders for Life-Sustaining Treatment). MOLST is a medical order form (similar to a prescription) that relays instructions between health professionals about a patient's care based on an individual's right to accept or refuse medical treatment, including treatments that might extend life. It is more detailed than a Do Not

Resuscitate order and, unlike an Advance Directive, can be put into effect as soon as it is signed and before the person becomes incapacitated.

Here are a few of the required documents, which are studded with an alphabet soup of medical abbreviations, most derived from Latin, such as PO (*per orem*) = by mouth; BID (*bis in die*) = twice a day; PRN (*pro re nata*) = as needed:

* Standing orders, the Fisher Home's normal medications, with dosages and frequency, listed under various categories of symptoms: mild to severe pain, dyspnea (difficulty with breathing), anxiety/agitation, nausea/vomiting, indigestion, excessive tracheal secretions, cough, skin issues, diarrhea, and constipation.

* Karnofsky Performance Status Scale, a standard for assessing a patient's capacities, with 100 representing normal and 10 signifying imminent death. In between are the numbers that represent a decline in function. For instance, 60 is described as "requires occasional assistance, but is able to care for most of his personal needs." Forty is "disabled, requiring special care and assistance."

* Lists of medical criteria for conditions that deter-

mine terminal prognosis. This is a crucial document for deciding whether a patient is eligible for admission to hospice and, later, whether that person continues to be eligible. A variety of conditions are listed, including stroke and coma, renal disease, pulmonary disease, cancer, and decline in clinical status. But lists of criteria are only guidelines, and, as each document states, "clinical judgment is required in each case."

ONCE THE NURSES AND OTHER STAFF members have completed their daily handwritten notes (the Fisher Home does not yet keep computerized records), all of this paperwork is carefully reviewed by two nurses designated as clinical managers and overseen by clinical director Kathy Curtis. It's a labor-intensive, ongoing process. The hospice must dot all the i's and cross all the t's in order to fulfill its license and be paid. And, of course, thanks to the nature of government bureaucracies, the regulations keep changing. Medicare has increased the number of its Additional Document Requests—supplemental material after the original documentation has been submitted. Kathy needs to keep on top of all those changes. The organization has to keep proving itself every day.

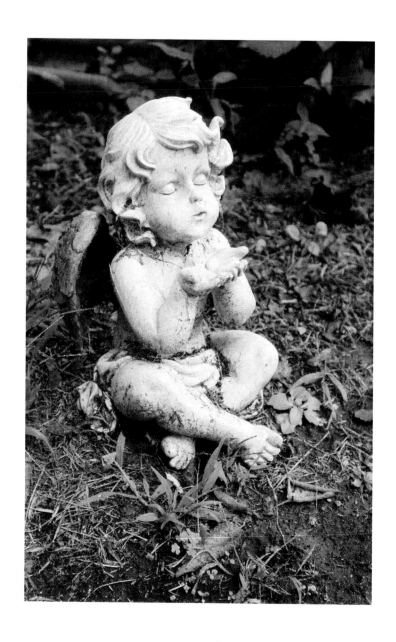

CHAPTER TEN

PRISCILLA WHITE:
WEAVING THE
HUMAN FABRIC

ONE OF THE FIRST PEOPLE a new patient at the Fisher Home will see, along with the attending nurse, is social worker Priscilla White. Priscilla is a gentle presence, with a low voice and a winning smile. She dresses unobtrusively in muted colors, her chin-length hair its own grayish-brown. She does not stand out in a crowd, yet there is no question that she can make herself heard when she needs to. She can be passionate about her principles, but she is also a rock of calm, practicality, and reason-ableness at the Fisher Home.

Priscilla has a history of making things happen in the community. A co-founder of Jessie's House, a local residence for homeless people and their families, she also worked at Grace House, an organization for addicted mothers. "This was when people were still dying of AIDS," recalls Priscilla. "It was just brutal for them to be dying, leaving those kids behind." Realizing that she wanted to stay in touch with end-of-life issues, she began her work with hospice, first in Greenfield's home hospice organization and then at the Fisher Home.

When someone arrives here, she does what's called a psycho-social assessment, which starts with a genogram, a chart of all the people in the family, several generations, living and dead, showing how they relate to the dying person, what they do or did, and where they live or lived. In hospice, she says, "We look at the whole system, rather than just one person." The genogram, which includes family friends as well as animals—dogs, cats, horses—helps staff and volunteers get a better picture of the person they are dealing with.

Priscilla often helps with people's practical concerns—how to help family members get transportation to the hospice, how to arrange for burials or find venues for memorial services. But like Norma Palazzo, she also tries to find out what sustains people in hard times. Sometimes people say it's their religion or their friends, and sometimes they mention their animals or their knitting or painting or writing poetry. "It's so open-ended that it's a wonderful bridge to building on the person's strength—which is why I love hospice so much," says Priscilla. This emphasis on the person's "whole system" is one of the ways hospice differs from the conventional medical model of care for a dying person. Looking at that whole system, says Priscilla, often indicates whether the patient is in one place—emotionally, psychologically—while family members are in another. Some family members may be denying that a loved one's end is near, while the patient is fully aware and accepting of that fact. The hospice team can establish a plan of care based on what they see as the strengths of each person.

Open-ended questions elicit the most helpful response, she finds. "Some people just talk about memories that make them feel they're part of their past. A ninety-six-year-old gentleman talked about that legacy," a legacy of tough German immigrants. One day when he was in pain, Priscilla let him know that he didn't have to suffer, that he could ask for medication. And he said, "I'm really able to tolerate it quite well." Priscilla got a sense that it was the legacy of those forebears that was sustaining him. He was feeling pain that he described as cutting and sharp, and yet he was deciding not to be medicated. "Honoring that decision is a very important part of respecting someone's choices, their dignity in making a good choice for themselves," she says. "It might not be the choice I would make, but that's the great thing about how we're all different." Hospice, she says, acknowledges that "there are so many ways of being in the world."

Families don't always agree with a patient's wishes. Sometimes they disagree among themselves about how to deal with the end of someone's life. Priscilla regularly talks with residents and family members about these ultimate concerns. Often she is able to help resolve conflicts. But if she and other staff members cannot help the family to an agreed-upon solution, she will turn to the hospice's ethics committee, a group she facilitates. That committee is composed of a physician, a psychologist, a minister, a lawyer, and clinical director Kathy Curtis. The group meets quarterly but can be convened at any time.

"We deal with issues—real cases from the Fisher Home—where it isn't clear how to go forward," says Priscilla. It's a chance to look at things from many points of view and helps clarify the next steps to be taken. There might be tension between the goals of the patient and family over what kinds of interventions to offer. When told about our dying friend Larry and his threats of suicide, Priscilla wonders whether the threats were real. "I've found in hospice over the years, we often hear people say things like: 'I don't want to live anymore; my life has no meaning; I can't bear all the losses I've had on so many levels.'" It's more about not being able to cope with the current situation. That's very different, she says, from wanting to commit suicide. That, she says, is where the hospice team can do an intervention.

She describes Larry's wife's stance as "resistance to the reality facing her and her husband. That resistance robs them of any chance to have a meaningful connection about this end stage of his life." She uses the paradigm of "alignment" when thinking about the Fisher Home's patients and their families. "Are the patient and the family in alignment with what is happening in the dying process or not? Do they want someone to eat who has gone beyond the ability to process food? Do they want someone to get up out of bed who is too debilitated to do it? Do they feel it is going too fast or too slowly?" Priscilla thinks this paradigm applies to how we live the rest of our lives: "Are we in alignment with what is, and able to go with it or not?"

All decisions at the Fisher Home, she says, refer back to the guiding ethical principles of hospice: autonomy, beneficence, nonmaleficence, and justice. The primary principle is autonomy: what does the patient want? An important addition is dignity—treating people as individuals, not as collections of symptoms—and a commitment to confidentiality.

Hospice has an arsenal of medications that can be used to alleviate pain, but they also reduce alertness—what's called the double effect. Sometimes patients choose not to alleviate much pain in order to maintain alertness. No one is forced to accept unwanted treatment. "Autonomy trumps anything else," says Priscilla. The next consideration, beneficence, refers to the effort to do good; and nonmaleficence is the embodiment of the physician's Hippocratic oath, *primum non nocere*—first of all, do no harm. Justice refers to the fair and equal treatment of all patients. Priscilla adds to these principles the values of truth and honesty. "Oftentimes, once everything is stated clearly, as honestly as possible, presented in a respectful, dignified way, people are able to get onto the same page and a lot of apparent discord resolves."

This is not to say that things are simple, even for experienced staff members, despite their ongoing training and practice in dealing with issues at the end of life. There are cultures and individual families in which death is not spoken of. In those cases, the hospice staff, as always, tries hard to respect the family's wishes. They may be asked, for instance, not to mention the word "hospice" in the presence of the patient, a request they have no trouble honoring.

And there are people who really do want to end their own lives. In Massachusetts, assisted suicide is illegal. A Death With Dignity law was voted down in a 2012 referendum. Physicians are not allowed to help people die, and hospice officially takes a stand against participating in any such action. Individual staff at the hospice may feel differently, but even if such a law were passed, the action to end a life would never be taken under hospice care. In fact, even in states where assisted suicide is legal, few patients request it.

In her private life Priscilla is a weaver, but it's easy to see her in that role as a professional as well. She describes the work of a residential hospice in the language of weaving: "You put up the warp—that's the long part—and you weave the weft through it." The warp is the hospice team, all the different threads and disciplines. And the weft is the patients and their families and friends, "a coming and going that changes every day—this beautiful weaving of the human spirit. The richness of it is the variation, very creative and unpredictable. We don't know who's going to be coming in the door and what that energy is going to bring into the Fisher Home."

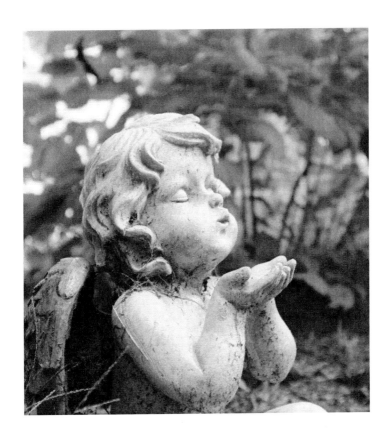

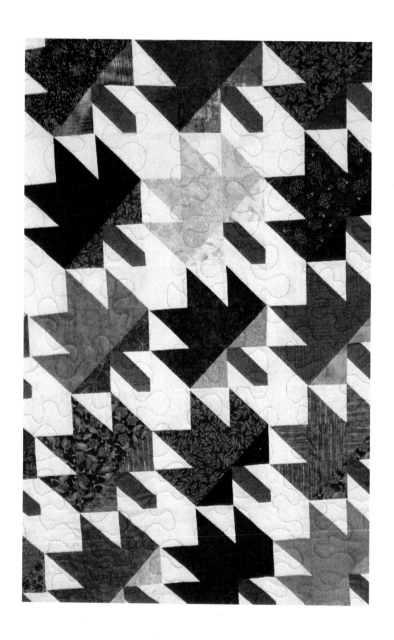

CHAPTER ELEVEN

LEE SHOTLAND:
PEACE AT LAST

WHEN LEE SHOTLAND DIED at age ninety-one, in June 2011, she had been at the Fisher Home for a year and a half, much longer than most of those who come there at the end of their lives. Often people come for only a few days. Currently the average stay is just under three weeks. Moving someone to a residential hospice is a difficult decision, and many people, both physicians and family members, often delay that move until the last possible moment. For hospice workers, such short stays are frustrating: not enough time to get to know the person, to understand his or her needs. A longer stay offers the chance to deliver the full range of hospice services—physical, emotional, spiritual, practical—and with it the hoped-for good death. Lee had been at the hospice long enough to be well known by both staff and volunteers. Even so, at the memorial service held at the hospice, there were genuine surprises. To begin with, about thirty-five people showed up, more than the most optimistic organizers would have expected. Then there were the reminiscences that showed she had created an unexpectedly affectionate legacy.

When Lee arrived at the hospice, she was angry and resentful of everything and everyone—the Parkinson's that was slowly draining her life away, the loss of her looks and energy, the people who were charged with her care, the food she was served, the way the world in general was going to hell in a handbasket. She held none of this back. As her youngest son, Jeff, describes her, not just then but throughout her life: "She was very passionate, loving, insecure, but at the same time a bold person, who tended to say what she thought without filtering at all."

In a first encounter with Lee, you might not have noticed the loving part in that string of adjectives. She tended to peer out suspiciously, like a witch in a fairy tale. She was loudly disapproving of C., a gentle resident with Alzheimer's, when he made a mess at the table. She complained about the food. "Could you eat that?" she'd ask, pointing to an innocuous piece of chicken in tomato sauce. "Would you make that at your house?" Speaking of someone's ex-wife, she said, "I always wondered where he picked up that bargain."

Yet at that memorial service, when people had a chance to look back, several volunteers described the satisfaction of feeling specially chosen for her affection. Lee had managed to create more than a few devoted friends, and there was almost a feeling of competition, of sibling rivalry in the room. A few recalled how Lee had reminded them of their own mothers, and how she had helped them come to terms with the memory of those sometimes difficult women. Volunteer Deb Gorlin told how her mother had never been reconciled to Deb's hair, a great halo of gray. She described a scene in which her mother, who was just coming out of anesthesia after surgery, took a look at Deb, who was leaning over her, and said: "Oh, my God, that hair!" Lee, on the other hand, had always been complimentary about Deb's hair. But Lee could also cast a sharp eye. Sometimes it came as a kind of backhanded tribute—"You look better today," she'd say—which left you wondering what you'd looked like last time.

Perhaps it was because her outlook was often so dark that when she said, "I'm always glad to see *you*," you felt specially favored.

Lee had had a hard life, growing up poor in New York State's rural Catskill region. It was an Orthodox Jewish household where Yiddish was spoken at home, although Lee and her five siblings were fluent in English. When Lee had children of her own, though they learned a few basic phrases, they were not encouraged to speak Yiddish, so it became the private language of the older generation. Lee's parents had moved upstate from Brooklyn, persuaded by an uncle that this farming community was heaven on earth. But Lee's father was not handy and had no agricultural skills. Jeff describes him as a cold, unfriendly man who never spoke. Both of Lee's parents were immigrants from small towns now in Ukraine. Both had had terrible early lives. Lee's father, whose own mother had died after being gored by a bull, was mistreated by his stepmother, kicked out of the house and made to live in a barn. Lee's mother believed that her own mother had—perhaps accidentally, perhaps not—poisoned her own husband. These were the dark shadows that hovered over Lee's childhood.

But she managed to get out. Though she was mostly a good student and, says Jeff, always "clever and insightful," she didn't finish high school because she couldn't get through algebra. College was not even a remote possibility. She and her two sisters moved to New York City, found work there, married, and stayed. She remained an urban person, says her middle son, Steve, who could remember nothing like taking walks with her in the woods. "A camper she was not," he says.

Lee married a businessman, and they moved to an apartment in Jamaica, Queens, a large multifamily building with some outdoor play space, as well as access to the apartments of friends and playmates for the three boys, who were born over the course of six years. Jeff describes this as a "tribal culture of about eight families, all with kids, all very blue-collar, working class." When they lived in Queens, he says, his mother had great friendships with some of the other families. It was "a very cohesive little microcommunity." She had a regular card game with a number of the women, a "girls' night out." Lee worked for her husband, who for a time had a lamp manufacturing business. Then she worked in a variety of secretarial and bookkeeping jobs. Being a working mother was unusual for a woman in those days, but Lee knew her family needed the extra money. Steve recalls that she was "both proud and put-upon" about her work.

In 1960, when Jeff, Steve, and Bruce were five, nine, and eleven, respectively, the family moved to Great Neck on Long Island, into what Jeff describes as a "fairly wealthy, upper-class Jewish, culturally sophisticated" environment. In Great Neck, the cohesive community vanished. Lee had a much harder time establishing friendships there, although she eventually did, despite what Jeff terms her "coarseness." Both sons describe a mother who always put her children first, giving them emotional support and tending to their physical needs. She was, says Steve, "a tiger mother and mother-in-law." She didn't have a lot of other, outside interests, and Steve remembers wishing that she'd had "more inner focus. She didn't know how to describe her emotional life." Bruce, the eldest, was the one who had the hardest time with his mom, describing their life-long relationship as "oil and water."

When the children were grown, Lee and her husband moved to Florida, where they lived for fifteen years. When her husband died, in 2002, Lee didn't want to stay there. She was then eighty-three and having difficulty walking. Along with this, says Steve, she was clinically depressed—she had stopped eating and was losing weight. At this point Jeff found an assisted living residence, the Arbors, in Amherst, just across the river from his household in Northampton. Lee lived there for ten years but never felt at home, never participated in any events, didn't dress, didn't take meals in the dining room, preferring to have them delivered to her room. Eventually Jeff hired some aides to help her out, especially at night. She'd had two episodes of falling when she'd refused to call for assistance, afraid of what was coming. As the youngest of six children, Lee had taken care of her siblings, often for months in their final illnesses. She feared a grim, long-drawn-out, painful end to her life. Says Jeff, "I used to have to shoot over there, sometimes more than once a week, to calm her down because she was sure she was about to die."

Before her husband's death, but especially afterward, Lee had been prone to panic attacks. Steve remembers the first one he encountered, while they were taking a walk in Washington, D.C. He was trying to tell her about his life. He needed to tell her that he was gay, and that he was "in a good place." But she couldn't deal with his coming out—she had to stop walking, had difficulty breathing. "She was locked in," he says. "She didn't have access to help, didn't discuss issues of concern."

At the Arbors, the panic increased, and the early symptoms of Parkinson's began to appear. It was her physician, Stephanie Osieki, who made the first contact with the Fisher Home. Dr. Osieki was amazing, says Steve, in the way she could connect with Lee. She went way beyond the call of duty, sometimes shopping for groceries, getting her chicken soup at Whole Foods. As Lee's condition deteriorated, Osieki recommended moving to the hospice, but Lee wasn't ready for it. Then, after a while, in a surprising move, Lee called the Fisher Home herself. "I'm ready," she said. "Come and get me." She didn't give up control, notes Steve. "She made the call, literally and figuratively." It was a huge relief to her sons.

From the day she moved to the Fisher Home, Steve says, she became more engaged, more involved. The first time he saw her there, she was dressed and had agreed to use a wheelchair, which made her much more mobile. She became more sociable and suffered no more anxiety attacks. She enjoyed being in the kitchen, folding laundry, watching a volunteer clean the fish tank, commenting on the proceedings. Jeff continued to visit regularly, and although Steve lives in San Francisco, he, too, became a regular presence for several days each month, taking his mother out for walks in her wheelchair, cooking special soups. When he worked in the kitchen, she would join him, watching and monitoring his every move. "You put parsley in at the beginning of the chicken soup? I never do that. What's that you're putting in now?" He took all this calmly, kept smiling as he cut up vegetables. It was clear, despite her carping, that Lee adored having him there, adored, too, the fact that he was cooking for her.

Despite the fact that she'd grown up in an Orthodox Jewish household and kept kosher much of her married life, Lee no longer insisted on any of these rules when she was at the Fisher Home. She was perfectly happy to eat a ham sandwich. In her last months of life, she spoke with a local rabbi, exchanging Yiddishisms with him in a pleasant encounter but not a deeply spiritual one. All three of her sons observed that the staff and volunteers attended not only to their mother's physical needs, but to her social needs as well. And all three felt at home there. Says Jeff, "You could go into the kitchen and help, or you could bring something to eat." Some of the aides at the time, Steve observes, were a little "rough around the edges," but Lee had no trouble speaking up for herself. Mainly, Jeff says, the staff was unusually talented in their combination of informality and responsibility, "making it feel like a family environment, something that's pretty hard to pull off." Now that Lee had twenty-four-hour care, Jeff was relieved of the burden of finding staffing to support his mother seven to eight hours a day, something he had been managing while she was at the Arbors. "It was a huge stressor," he says. "People didn't show up. I had to fight with the agency."

Says Bruce, "Overall, I would rate the Fisher Home a 12 out of 10 in terms of how it affected the end of Mom's life. It truly became her 'home,' even in her own words. The compassion of everyone who works there is amazing to me and will always be. These are people who love humanity and show it each and every day; they talk the talk, but also walk the walk."

Until the very end, her family remained at the center of Lee's life. She continued to enjoy her grandchildren, Jeff's children, who visited her at the Fisher Home and were there the day she died. Jeff had seen a real change in Lee's way of dealing with her sons during her final months—"certain things like not bringing up how upsetting my separation from my wife was for her." Holding back like that would have been impossible for her before, Jeff believes. This change made their relationship much easier: "We could really enjoy each other's company in a way that was hard to do before. In the past, she'd always throw in those zingers."

At the memorial celebration, held in the hospice's dining room, spiritual counselor Norma Palazzo opened with a Jewish prayer. Lee's three sons spoke about their mother and about how grateful they were to the Fisher Home for making the end of her life so peaceful and pleasant both for her and for them. She was not an easy character, they agreed, but something about this place had softened her, allowed her to rest in peace at last, even before her final departure. They were humorous and affectionate, telling little anecdotes about her—a mother who, despite her sharp edges, had been the source of an absolutely unconditional love. They had brought food—bagels and lox and other ethnically appropriate items to be shared after the service.

When people were invited to reminisce, they recalled how Lee liked to have her feet rubbed, how she enjoyed arranging flowers, how she always commented on people's appearance, how she had an opinion on pretty much everything. Then came the revelations about how many people thought Lee saw them as special friends. If there was any sentimentalizing of this often cranky and difficult woman, it was overborne by the frank depiction of a real person, a strong woman with genuine struggles, who fought to retain her humanness to the end.

When he first visited the Fisher Home, Jeff reminisced, he wasn't sure it was the right place: "It seemed almost *too* homey." He wasn't sure it offered the security of an institution; it seemed too small. It took him a few months to be convinced. The proof was in how Lee felt. "She blossomed," he said, "found a part of herself that she'd lost. She felt she wasn't being judged in a negative way, that she was being given the benefit of the doubt. I think she felt comfortable in her skin for the first time since she lived in Queens, where she had a group of soul mates. Here she had soul mates again. It was kind of a miracle to end up that way. My brothers and I want to reserve a place there."

Very quiet day. Gent here for respite
has gone home; Isabel out to lunch
with her daughter; L. very quiet after
a walk up and down the hall; E.'s family here to visit; only C. needs my
help with lunch. He is his old cheerful self. Now getting all food ground
up to prevent choking. Some coughing,
despite that.

   I learn that not everyone who comes
to hospice has a Do Not Resuscitate
order. Surprises me. Why would you
agree to hospice care and then want to
be brought back? Sometimes it's family
members who don't want to let nature
take its course. But sometimes, I
learn, people arrive having just found
out about a terminal diagnosis and
need time and help to come to terms
with their approaching death.

***

Lots of the time volunteering is just
a kind of game of chance. W., whose
daughter comes every day to feed her
and give her one of her three gin and
tonics, is hard to visit, partly
because of her daughter's heavy presence, and partly because she is very
deaf, not to mention old--ninety-six,
and sleeping a lot. L., a charming
lady I met just the other day, was

asleep, and a new resident who can
only be fed by relatives or staff is
also sound asleep. I help a little in
the kitchen, clearing out dishes, putting away pots and pans, but it sure
feels desultory.

***

Gerard has had unsettling news about
problems with his daughter's preg-
nancy. She is four and a half months
along. Priscilla had been talking with
him for about two hours. She thinks he
might like some company. I wait a
while and go in, make a little small
talk. Do I like "M*A*S*H," he asks--
he's known to love it. I never watched
it much in its heyday of the 1970s,
but am happy to give it a try. So we
watch a few episodes, both of us laughing loudly at this broad and slightly
risqué comedy about medics during the
Korean War. A pleasant interlude. We
do not talk about his daughter.

***

New resident, C., takes me on photo tour
of Holy Land, makes me want to visit
Petra, ancient city carved from sand-
stone cliffs--relation to New Mexico
native people?

Z. is moaning, wailing. I comfort
her, talk, stroke her arm. She calms
down, tells me she "misses her relatives." These are not the nieces, who
live at a distance, but the ones who
are gone, dead. She dozes a minute,
then wakes and says, "Can I have some
candy?" I try to oblige but fail to find
any. She's not interested in ice cream.
We watch some figure skating on TV.

***

Felix Oppenheim has arrived. His wife,
Shulamith, is here, very distraught.
I have been slightly acquainted with
both of them over the years in Amherst.
She goes off to lunch, and I sit with
Felix, a distinguished political scientist, who is blind and ninety-eight.
He has fallen and shattered his femur.
He does not speak, but can indicate
yes and no. Refuses painkiller from
nurse, accepts liquidy mouth swab from
me. I sit and stroke his arm, then
read the paper, sing a few old French
songs. Shulamith has told me they
speak only French with each other.
It's a sixty-three-year marriage. "He
is on his last journey and I cannot go
with him," she says. She tells me a
bit of his eventful life story: He was
in the Belgian army, captured by Nazis,

escaped Europe via Portugal, then
drafted into U.S. Army.

As I leave the building, a birthday
party for T. is not getting under way.
He has refused to get up. Norma has
organized a cake and card and gift
(a truck of some sort).

***

Halloween snow disaster has come and
gone. Fisher Home survives nicely
because generator working well. My
house still has no power. I come here
to warm up.

Q. is here, dying of a brain disease. His sister is one of my tennis-
playing friends. She's predictably
strong, but very sad. We talk, then
hug. When I see her at tennis, she
asks when I'll be at the hospice next.
I send her an e-mail with my hours.

***

Talk at length with Q.'s wife, who is
waiting for the doctor to discuss what
to do with her husband's body after
his death. A university medical school
wants it for autopsy of his brain, and
the family agrees, but a doctor has to
sign papers for funeral home--Douglass,
here in town. She wants to make sure.

She is mostly matter-of-fact, but also
breaks down a little.

***

I visit T., who is sitting in his
lounger, leaning forward, groaning,
Oh, oh, oh. Hi, I say. How are you
doing? Not good, he says. In pain? I
ask. No pain, he says. Aide says he's
been very grouchy, wouldn't let her
near him. So I sit for a while, not
saying much. There's a tray with
mostly uneaten breakfast--scrambled
eggs with mushrooms, buttered toast,
cold coffee. He bolts down a little
toast, and I ask what he'd really
like. "Some of that," pointing to the
eggs. I make him a couple of fresh
scrambled eggs and new toast (no jam!)
and heat up the coffee. He eats most
of it. "I can't remember anything," he
says. So I remind him of some things
that he has remembered, using photos
in the room--his wife, his grandkids,
him in a truck. Move the lounger so
that he can have his feet up and head
back a little. Then he calls for the
aide to help him go to the bathroom--
Quick!" he says.
  As I pass J.'s room, she tells me
she's dropped a picture on the floor and
broken the glass. I get her to sit back

down, find a broom, and clean that up.

In the hall, a member of Eventide, an a capella group that sings for people who are dying. Could I find out who wants to listen, who might like to have them come to the room? I do a little canvass and get N. and S. into the living room, where the group sings beautifully. Another regular musical contributor is Barbara Russell, who comes with her Celtic harp to sit at people's bedsides, if they wish. Her music is soothing, ethereal, nonspecific, more like breathing than singing.

***

When I arrive, Jenn tells me that T. died just a few minutes ago. According to Ilsa's note later in the day, one of the aides was massaging his feet when he expired. Soon afterward, his daughter invited the staff into the room to say some prayers and to reminisce, a nice gesture.

In the kitchen I meet up with J.'s daughter, looking distraught and exhausted. J. is not dying fast enough, and there is conflict among the daughters about who is putting in enough time. I mention my experience with my mother's long, slow death and

suggest that some people just don't
agree to let go. I offer her something
to eat and we settle on a grilled
cheese sandwich on pumpernickel. I
slice an orange on the plate, like a
not very good restaurant.   ,

***

Spend part of my seventy-fifth birthday
helping clean out the hospice's
garage. Jenn has arranged for a dumpster, and it is already partly filled
when I get there in the afternoon.
Grant Milner, one of the volunteers,
is there with his truck, hauling big
items. He is probably about my age--
a vet, cheerful, energetic, and effective. It is pouring, the area between
the driveway and the dumpster quickly
turning into a mudhole. I put a few
boards down to make a path, then we
happily toss stuff. Out goes the
decaying lumber alongside the building, along with broken pieces of furniture. Some usable stuff goes to the
Hospice Shop. Extra commodes, walkers,
and wheelchairs to the Belchertown
senior center. I head home to take a
shower and get ready for my birthday
dinner out.

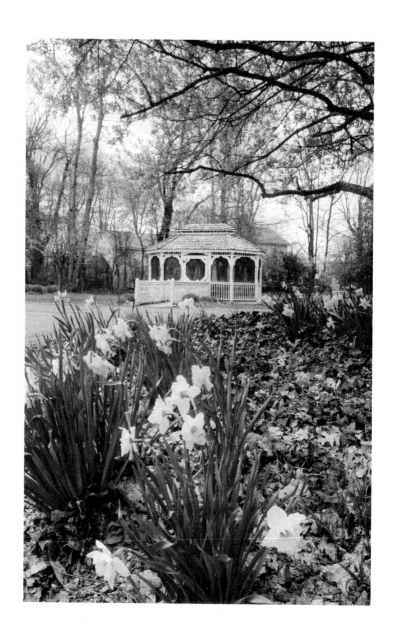

CHAPTER 12

ILSA MYERS:
PROBLEM SOLVER,
MATCHMAKER

Ilsa Myers, the Fisher Home's volunteer coordinator, has the gift of making places feel attractive and inviting. This is a crucial skill in a residential hospice, a place that aims to be as homelike as possible in order to normalize the experience of dying and provide an alternative to the noisy, high-stress atmosphere of a modern hospital. Ilsa's own home is large and eclectically furnished, an old farmhouse with wraparound porches, several parlors, and a big, well-used kitchen. When hospice volunteers meet there, she can provide enough chairs for most of us, and she has baked cookies and fruit breads to keep our stomachs content while we discuss issues of life and death, spirit and body. At the Fisher Home she has managed to make her tiny windowless office into a cozy place to sit and talk. She enjoys these exchanges, and that's important, because it represents a lot of what she does as volunteer coordinator. "I love that," she says. "I'm a networker, I love to connect."

Ilsa brings enormous energy and cheerfulness to a job that is a cross between mother superior, confidante, and traffic cop. A problem solver who sees difficulties as opportunities, she is a vivid presence, with curly gray hair, dressed in original combinations of ethnic-looking vests, muted scarves, and draped sweaters, some of them her own creations.

Before coming to the Fisher Home, Ilsa worked as a hospice volunteer in people's homes. Here, she sees herself, in part, as a "matchmaker." She gets to know residents' wishes and needs, then tries to connect them with compatible volunteers. She'll say, "Denise, our resident in Room Four is a pianist. You might try to find out what kind of music she likes to listen to." Or, "Jim has been talking about going out to get corn on the cob. Could you drive him to the farm stand on Pine

Street?" Sometimes, when residents have asked to be left alone, it's a matter of reminding volunteers to keep their distance. "Don't go in unless Susan rings, and only long enough to find out what she needs and maybe bring her a cup of tea." Sometimes she'll look for specific pairings: a Buddhist to spend time with someone who wants to find serenity, a gardener who can talk about raising vegetables, a cat lover.

Ilsa has a hearty laugh that you can hear all the way down the hall from her office. Describing herself as "somewhat of a Pollyanna," someone who likes to see people succeed, she is ebullient and optimistic, but also firm in upholding hospice principles. One of those principles involves helping volunteers learn to set boundaries. Don't bring your problems to the hospice, says Ilsa. "Leave your stuff in the car. You had a difficult morning; your son is struggling. If you're not really ready to come in and leave your son's story in the car, it's probably not a good day to come." Volunteers need to be focused on the hospice.

Emotional boundaries also need to be established. Some volunteers may become overinvolved, neglecting their own families or becoming resentful when a resident's family doesn't take their advice. At such moments Ilsa may need to take the volunteer aside for a reminder to step back.

Twice a year Ilsa runs seven-week classes for prospective volunteers. Before they begin, she screens applicants to try to identify and weed out people who are especially needy or others who just want "something to do." It would be a waste of everyone's time, she says, to go through the application process, have them write an essay, and check their references, "knowing full well that by the second class, that person is going to realize that this is not really for them." She looks for people whose lives are "so rich and satisfactory that they want to give back. Sometimes they've had a wonderful experience with hospice." She believes that there is a calling to this kind of work. Hospice volunteers should feel proud, she says, "because you are putting yourself into a situation that many people wouldn't want to be in. They will say, 'Oh, I don't know how you do it.'"

Like others who work in the Fisher Home and most who work with hospice, Ilsa has her own attitudes about death and dying. Her cheerful temperament extends to those attitudes. "Dying," she says, "is as natural as birthing. I feel we should fear death no more than we fear life."

I'm reading Julian Barnes' memoir
"Nothing to be Frightened Of," centered
on his witty and wise meditations on
death. I keep wanting to copy things
down. Here's one bit, as he considers
the question of what we fear more,
death or dying:

> Almost everyone fears one to the exclusion
> of the other; it's as if there isn't enough
> room for the mind to contain both. If you
> fear death, you don't fear dying; if you fear
> dying, you don't fear death. But there's no
> logical reason why one should block out the
> other; no reason why the mind, with a lit-
> tle training, cannot stretch to encompass
> both. As one who wouldn't mind dying as
> long as I didn't end up dead afterwards, I
> can certainly make a start on elaborating
> what my fears about dying might be.*

***

Christmas Eve Day spent at the hospice
making food for the future--a couple
of quiches and a big pot of chili,

---

* Julian Barnes, *Nothing to Be Frightened Of* (New York: Knopf, 2008), 137.

all to freeze in small quantities.

One of the aides and I talk about husbandly gift mistakes. Hers gave her some sexy lingerie one year (not comfortable!!), and mine gave me a heavy flannel nightie (I,like to sleep in silk). Neither one was paying attention. Last year he gave her some nice-looking scrubs and a new pair of sneakers. Just right.

The place is too quiet, too few residents, not enough work needing to be done. This is the rhythm of hospice, all or nothing.

**

Quieter still on New Year's Eve Day-- only three residents. One is D., whose feet I rub for a while, which she enjoys. She tells me her views of the afterlife. She is Catholic, and likes occasionally getting communion here from her local priest. She thinks "what comes next" is "whatever He has planned for me." She is cheerful, content in her beliefs.

Staff considering whether they can accommodate a 500-pound woman in end stage of congestive heart failure, whose doc wants to send her here.

A new challenge. The house's Hoyer
lift is good for 250 pounds. They'd
have to get a new, bigger one and
always have two aides on duty. A different bed, too? One aide tells me she
has taken care of a hugely obese
patient but someone who was able to
walk on her own. A very different situation. This person will probably not
last more than a few days--but who
knows? She is in a hospital, where
they have equipment and staff to deal
with her. The hospice ends up not
accepting her.

***

Z. is having many weepy periods. One
nurse believes this can be handled by
human contact. That has been my experience: When she's crying, I come in
and hold her hand and talk to her. She
will usually calm down pretty quickly
and usually goes to sleep after that.
But the weepy jags are getting more
frequent and other nurses are in favor
of using medication to calm her--small
amounts would work, it seems. This is
a real clinical/philosophical difference. When and how and how much to
medicate, and for what?

B. dies while I am on my shift. As
she usually does after a death, Ilsa
sends out an e-mail to all volunteers:

"B., in Room 6, died at 12:20 this
afternoon, surrounded by his wife and
children. . . a particularly devoted
family who deeply appreciated their
stay with us. Thank you all for
another good ending."

Now only four residents out of a pos-
sible nine. This low number is a real
problem for the hospice financially.
Kathy says they are getting referrals,
it's just that they haven't worked out.
People die or make different choices.
They are cooperating well with Cooley
Dickinson Hospital, she says.

***

State Department of Public Health officials have been here for a couple of
days making an assessment. The two
ladies want to interview a volunteer,
so I oblige. They ask, among other
things, what I understand hospice to
be. They seem surprised that I have
thought about this. Ask what I think
of the staff and I give everyone an A
for skill and devotion. Everyone here
a little nervous about their presence,

but the ladies express lots of admiration for the place. I tell them it is
where I'd be happy to die, and they
nod approvingly.

Tally volunteer hours for Ilsa with
a calculator, long columns of numbers.
Then sit with Z. while she spoons in
her ground-up chicken, rice, and
pureed green veg. Asked if she'd like
dessert. Yes, of course. I bring chocolate ice cream with chocolate sauce.

* * *

Our old friend Howard Ziff died this
morning. Jane, his wife, was here
overnight, as she has been for the
past few days. She said, "It will be
my last chance to spend any nights
with him." Her son and daughter are
here, son from California, daughter
from the Netherlands.

Howard had had a crisis of congestive heart failure at the university
swimming pool. They had him in the
intensive care unit for several days,
saying that only open heart surgery
could help, but that he too fragile to have it. Plus all the dementia.
So hospice. But he was extremely agi-
tated, and almost the first thing the

family was told was that if the Fisher
Home couldn't handle him, they might
have to send him somewhere else, perhaps back to the hospital. With a
small staff, the hospice can't keep
people they can't'control and who
might hurt themselves or others. But
I assured the family that the Fisher
Home would make every effort to calm
him down--meaning medication, among
other things. And the family made it
clear that that was what they wanted.
He could no longer speak for himself.

So that was a problem for Lucy, the
nurse, to get enough of the right
meds--a big guy, absorbing a lot--from
docs who are hard to reach on the
weekend. Before they found the right
meds, I'd sat on the side of the bed
with him while the family went out to
lunch. It was a bit of a wrestling
match to keep him from getting his
legs out over the side. Beds at the
Fisher Home have only partial railings. More railings would constitute
restraints, Lucy explained, although
the patient can agree to them, if he
is able, and a health care proxy can
also make that decision.

***

Ilsa is working with a volunteer who
doesn't want to do anything except
have "meaningful conversations" with
residents, not just sit with the
dying. Ilsa explains that volunteers
need to be available for pretty much
anything. Not all residents are up for
meaningful, or even any, conversation.
There's always the laundry to fold and
the dishes to wash.

***

The resident census has picked up
quite a bit since the drought of the
holidays and after, maybe partly a
result of some serious efforts on
behalf of the management crew. Priscilla, Ilsa, Norma are reaching out to
social workers at Bay State Medical
Center in Springfield, putting an
announcement of sponsorship on public
radio, nicely designed ads in appropriate publications.

***

I'm practicing my Spanish with Q.,
who is dying of some kind of cancer

that has invaded his liver. He is
quite yellow. He recently married his
longtime partner, E., who is here most
of the time. She speaks pretty good
English, cooks his favorite dishes, of
which he's not eating much. On the
stove are two pots, one with beans,
the other with a cornmeal and salt cod
mixture. She gives me a taste, very
good. She's spunky and able to be
cheerful, even while showing me photos
of him from a few months ago--hefty
and healthy. He tells me he has two
sons in Mexico and that he worked in
tobacco here in the valley.

***

A "Viennese Tea" at the Lord Jeff Inn
for hospice and Hospice Shop volunteers. Ilsa in her glory, having organized a successful event once again
with Hospice Shop director Ali Diamond. Celtic harpist Barbara Russell
plays in the corridor, and Eventide is
singing in the room where we gather.
About eighty people attending, 99 percent women, average age sixty-five. In
the corner of the big room, a table
full of classy-looking sweets, in
which we are invited to indulge after

the speeches. A brief introduction by
Ilsa, then more somber words from
Norma, a brief greeting from Kathy,
then a cheery, enthusiastic one from
Shauneen Kocot, new head of the home's
board. Shauneen, wearing a light tur-
quoise linen suit, stands up and puts
on a hat covered with artificial flowers, explaining that she'd spotted it
a while ago at the Hospice Shop and
just couldn't resist. She speaks about
coming to visit her mother-in-law,
Dot, every day during her eleven-month-
long stay at the hospice residence,
praising the staff in nice detail--
teakettle on the boil for her, coffee
waiting for her husband, Peter,
incredibly attentive care for Dot, who
was always perfectly clean and sweet
smelling. She makes us all feel good
about what we are doing.

Eventide serenades us, and we join
in with "You Are My Sunshine." We are
thanked for our volunteer contribu-
tions and head home. Outside, the
Extravaganja Festival--Amherst's annual
celebration of legalizing marijuana--
is in full swing. You could float home
on a contact high.

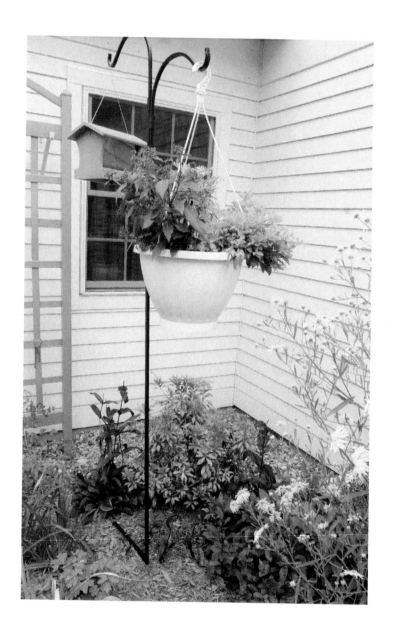

CHAPTER THIRTEEN

ISABEL GLASS:
A LONG, FULL LIFE

O NE OF THE RESIDENTS with whom Lee Shotland had a strong but sometimes scratchy relationship was Isabel Glass, another long-term resident and, like Lee, a Parkinson's sufferer. Unlike Lee, whose early years had been ones of poverty and struggle, Isabel had led a privileged life. She had been a writer and editor for fashion magazines, a doctor's wife who traveled widely and enjoyed art and literature. Lee would occasionally make cutting comments about Isabel's appearance or her willingness to eat whatever was put on the table. It sounded like resentment, but Lee's son, Jeff, interprets the behavior differently. He thinks she was intimidated: "It was a clash of cultures." But there was an overlap, too. Both of them had lived in New York, and, says Margot Glass, Isabel's daughter, Isabel liked Lee, even "identified with her a little."

Isabel lived at the Fisher Home almost as long as Lee did. Both women, having endured a slow, difficult decline, were more than ready for the end when it came. But their earlier lives were worlds apart. Born in the upper-middle-class Boston suburb of Brookline, Isabel graduated from Goucher College and moved to New York shortly afterward. She worked at an art gallery and later as a copywriter at fashion magazines, including *Harper's Bazaar*. She married a physician who specialized in cardiovascular disease, and had two daughters, one of whom died at a year old. A writer of fiction, she published two novels, one about a hospital, the other about the fashion world. The hospital novel, *Bedside Manners*, translated into several languages, is described on the cover as "a shockingly candid novel about the private lives—and loves—behind the big city hospital scene."

Isabel, who had had an apartment in a local independent living community, arrived at the Fisher Home after a stay in a nursing home, which had followed several hospitalizations. "She had bounced around from the hospital to rehab facility to another rehab/nursing home for several months," says her daughter. Isabel was exhausted, frightened, and depressed, and had decided she wanted to be taken to the hospice. She had been declining rapidly during those weeks and months, and it became clear, says Margot, that "she was not going to rebuild skills to return to the level of independent living" that had existed before all the hospitalization and rehabilitation. A few days after her mother arrived at the hospice, Margot asked her how she was feeling, and Isabel replied, "I feel like I've had all the bones in my body removed. I haven't been this relaxed in so long. I finally feel comfortable." She could now accept that she'd reached a point in her illness where, says Margot, "she didn't have to worry about pretending to be well or fighting to run away from it. She was exhausted and had made her peace with it. She was ready for everybody else to acknowledge that."

At the hospice, she found people to talk with about how she felt. Recalls Margot, "Anyone that she reached out to made themselves available to her." Isabel told her daughter that she'd been doing a lot of reading and talking, and that she felt ready. She had lived a good life, had eaten in the best restaurants, had good friends, traveled, read good books. "My mother had lived a very long, full life, and had never been afraid to face anything. I was so relieved to see her enter a place where everything was normalized, comfortable, and positive, and each day everybody met her exactly where she was at, however that was, without any judgment."

One of the staff whom Isabel especially appreciated was CNA team leader Jenn Messinger. As Margot puts it, "Jenn had kind of a little bit of an acerbic, funny wit. It was very secure, because it was so clear there was affection and true compassion behind it. My mother and she would have little play fights, like if my mother was refusing to eat something she'd asked Jenn to make." They'd kind of bicker, says Margot, but in a loving way. "I felt like that was great because it offset the softness of the general tone. She was so strong and direct with her."

"Normalizing" death is a big part of what hospice tries to do. In our culture, where the word cannot be spoken in public and often not even in private, putting death in its proper place is a difficult task. It involves undoing the habits of lifetimes. Still, for Isabel and her family—Margot, her husband, Pablo Yglesias, and their son and daughter—seeing death as a continuation of life was both comforting and strengthening.

Nevertheless, calm acceptance was not possible at every step along the way. Isabel was often frustrated and depressed by the loss of her abilities as her decline stretched out inexorably over the course of more than a year. She enjoyed reading and being read to, and she enjoyed her conversations with volunteers, especially those who shared her interest in the arts and who sympathized with her leftish politics. But she was becoming less able to enjoy even the more sedentary activities. Eventually, says Margot, "She couldn't really hear very well; she couldn't see the screen to watch a movie; she was getting a little fuzzy so that sometimes it was hard for her to follow a plot; she was having trouble with her breathing. She would say, 'I'm here and I accept that,' but it was hard sometimes."

As it is for many people at the end of life, food was tremendously important to Isabel, and in the beginning, Margot and Pablo would take her out for sushi or bring in things they knew she would enjoy. After having been on a pureed diet at the nursing home, where she had been choking, she took considerable pleasure in being able to eat normal food at the hospice and being able to ask for what she wanted. That didn't mean she didn't complain about the food at times, but here she knew she could ask for what she wanted and someone would make the effort to get it for her, even if it was just an egg and some juice. As Margot puts it, "It wasn't just tepid food on plastic plates on a gray tray that had been sitting in the hall on a trolley for forty-five minutes."

Isabel loved the weekends when volunteeer George Maston would make breakfast for those residents who were still able to enjoy them. George would bring his own pots and pans and ingredients, and prepare special omelets and other foods, to be served on trays in people's rooms or in the dining room if they were able to get there. Remembering Isabel's preferences, George says he would often make her a fresh fruit plate with mango, papaya, and cherries, plus a freshly baked chocolate or almond croissant, "foods that weren't often found at the Fisher Home." Some other favorites were anything with hollandaise sauce—a variation of eggs Benedict with smoked salmon and dill hollandaise.

Some of Isabel's best times at the Fisher Home were

spent at the piano, which she had studied when young, then returned to as an adult. She could be heard practicing Poulenc's "Mouvements Perpétuelles" and Debussy's "Children's Corner," but the majority of her playing was devoted to a whole range of old-time popular and Broadway tunes—Cole Porter, Rodgers and Hart, Gershwin, "Begin the Beguine," "Smoke Gets in Your Eyes," "Stardust." She had all these tunes and their lyrics in her head and under her hands. It was a pleasure to hear her play, to sit with her, suggest songs, and sing along with them. When Isabel was at the piano, her Parkinsonian tremors almost disappeared.

Margot feels that, paradoxically, her mother's life opened up when she came to the hospice—at a point, she notes, when many people's lives narrow and they become more isolated. Isabel connected with a lot of people, and the connection went both ways. Margot was especially impressed with how "graceful" the volunteers were, approaching people they didn't know yet—seeming to understand "how not to intrude, how to make the overture and respect the uncertainty of it." She remembered one time when her mother was getting confused and thinking Margot was *her* mother, and one of the volunteers came over to her and asked,

"What kind of a day are you having, Isabel?" Margot thought it was the perfect thing to say because it was, in fact, the big question.

Priscilla, the social worker, was great with her, says Margot. "Isabel and Priscilla did a lot of work together: what it all meant, what Isabel's concerns were, and how to resolve them—or not—and be comfortable with *not* having certain things resolved, if that was the case." One of the good things about the place, Margot thinks, was the variety of personalities. On any given day, "depending on what my mother felt up for, she could connect with a different person."

At a certain point, Isabel could no longer talk on the phone, even though they tried headsets and other arrangements. So Margot began spending more time at the hospice, up to five days a week. Finally, with Priscilla and Ilsa's help, she extricated herself a little. She knew she needed to make the transition, "but it was hard, because there was so much going on, and being there felt right. It wasn't that I worried that she wasn't getting enough care, it was just a feeling that we couldn't communicate any other way." She wanted to make sure her mother didn't feel "dumped."

The walls of Isabel's room at the Fisher Home held

a gallery of family pictures, framed and matted, many of them from generations past, chosen to reflect a history that Isabel could present to the world like a work of art, unlike the usual informal photos found in other residents' rooms, out-of-focus shots of barbecues or holiday gatherings. Such visual presentations mattered to Isabel. She cared about her personal appearance, and in the early days of her stay at the hospice would go out shopping for clothes at local discount outlets with her daughter. She could look chic in anything. Even at the very end, when she was tiny and diminished, she would appear in the living room looking elegant in an ocelot-patterned shirt and khaki pants.

Because of the care she and her family got at the Fisher Home, says Margot, "I was able to grieve and process a lot of it while my mother was still alive. I felt I almost front-loaded my grieving." Afterward, she didn't feel the need to take part in bereavement groups, although she did touch base with Norma a few times. But her son Isaac wanted to go back to the Fisher Home, because while his grandmother was there, he said, "I always thought of it as a place where I liked to see her, where we felt at home, and I don't now want to think of it as a bad place." So they went back and visited with

Norma for about half an hour, and that felt like closure for Isaac, says Margot. "He wanted to remember that it was a safe and good place, that it was OK that she wasn't alive anymore. He felt really comforted being able to sit with Norma."

Margot recalls a few times when the hospice staff stepped in to anticipate her family's needs. They told her that arrangements could be made for her to stay in the room with her mother overnight. Margot said no, her mother had never wanted roommates: "She and I were so close, but I don't think it would be fair to her. And I'm trying to accept that it's time for her to go." Then, a couple of days before Isabel died, one of the volunteers was sitting with her, holding her hand, and Margot remembers that nurse Lucy Fandel came in and, in an uncharacteristically short tone, asked Margot to step outside. Lucy was worried that this volunteer, however well intentioned, could be detracting from an important time. If Margot felt it as an intrusion, Lucy would ask the volunteer to leave. Margot said it was an important friendship, and it was fine. But, she added, "If she stays all day, I'll give you a signal."

Isabel died the night of February 20, 2011. She was eighty-four. June Bishop, the aide, was with her, holding her hand. The next morning, Margot and Pablo said to Isaac and his sister Nona, "You don't have to come if you feel you don't want to be there." They had already seen how much Isabel had changed in her final days. "She was always my mother until the very last minute," says Margot, "but in the last week, she became a kind of universal dying human. It wasn't frightening, it was just something that was bigger than her personality." The grandkids felt it wasn't fair for their parents to decide whether they should see their grandmother after her death. Isaac said, "Please don't tell me what I can't handle."

That morning, Margot remembers, was a "beautiful, calm, blue-sky day, really peaceful and clear." She was grateful that her children were able to be there with them, and come and go, and kiss their grandmother, and not be afraid to touch her. It felt peaceful and very natural.

At a memorial service at the Poets House in lower Manhattan in May, three months after her mother's death, Margot spoke about Isabel, her lifelong love of the arts and the wide range of her friendships, which continued to grow throughout her life. She spoke about her love of family, and how much pleasure she took from hearing her grandchildren make music, and how encouraging Isabel had always been of Margot's own path as an artist.

Isabel had traveled widely, something she continued to do even after her diagnosis. At the Fisher Home, a month before she died, she spoke to Margot about going on a trip with her aunt Fannie, a favorite relative who was no longer alive. Hospice workers report that it is not uncommon for people to speak this way in their last days. Some interpret it as a metaphor for the final trip out of life. Whatever its meaning, Margot was happy that her mother was anticipating a pleasant journey with someone she cared about.

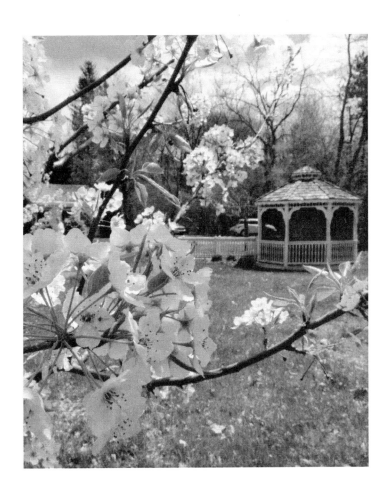

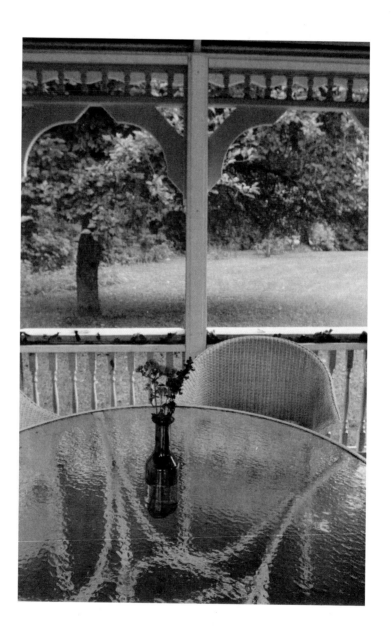

CHAPTER FOURTEEN

JENN MESSINGER:
WHAT SHE'D WANT
FOR HERSELF

J ENN MOVES FAST. She's down the hall to answer a resident's call bell before you can turn around. Cleaning up the kitchen takes no time, nor does putting together a meal for six residents, all of whom have different needs and tastes. Her directions to a volunteer or another aide are clear: Sam gets cranberry juice, and remember to put in a scoop of Thick-It, a thickening powder; Janet's food has to be pureed, and she doesn't like broccoli, so cook her some peas. Here's the tray with Francine's lunch. She'll need help eating it. Jenn can show a nice wiseguy sense of humor and doesn't take herself too seriously, but she is altogether serious about her job and about how her co-workers do theirs. At the same time, she's unfailingly warm and compassionate toward the residents.

She remembers one inveterate pipe smoker who sat outside in the covered entryway in all kinds of weather. People have been able to have their glass of wine or their gin and tonic. "They've always done it," says Jenn, "and they should be doing it here. They should be doing everything they like to do and enjoying the last part of their lives. I would want it that way for myself."

Jenn is a certified nurse's assistant, with additional certification as a hospice and palliative care nursing assistant. Well before earning those certifications, she had her first job, her first paycheck at age sixteen as an aide in a nursing home. At the Fisher Home, she has moved up the ranks to become the team leader of all the CNAs—usually referred to simply as aides. These are the people who have the most basic and intimate physical contact with residents—bathing them, repositioning them in bed, changing their incontinence briefs, preparing their food and feeding them. Nurses, who are charged with all the medical aspects of patient care, will help with these tasks, but the responsibility for what are known as activities of daily living—hygiene, mobility, nutrition, grooming, toileting—

belongs to the aides. Their skill, positive outlook, and good humor are crucial to the emotional welfare of residents and their families.

Jenn learned the importance of a caregiver's attitude when her uncle was dying. She was working in the nursing home at the time, and she could see that the care her uncle got in his own home was unlike anything she was seeing in her workplace. The people attending to him weren't hospice certified, she remembers, but "they just did this wonderful thing with him. It was unbelievable how they talked to him and how they approached him." The aide would watch for changes in his condition, and was reassuring and loving both to him and to the family, explaining that he didn't have to eat if he didn't feel like it, that they shouldn't force food or liquids on him. That marked a turning point for Jenn. She began doing private duty with people who were dying. "The nursing home," she says, "was good for certain things—for rehab, for activities—but for dying, definitely not." She came to believe that all of us need somebody to be with us at the end of our lives. We and our families shouldn't go through this process alone. In nursing homes, she observes, "Too many people die by themselves."

At the Fisher Home, Jenn spends time on the floor, dressed in scrubs and sneakers, doing an aide's work—fixing meals, doing the laundry, but most importantly tending to patients' needs. When she arrives in the morning, she gets the report from the overnight aide, then checks in on all the patients. After that, she says, "I do my temperatures." This is a state requirement, making sure that the residence's refrigerators are cold enough to keep food safe and that the water temperature is not so hot that it could injure someone. She talks to the nurses to see what their ideas are for the day. When she works with Sharon Kemp, another aide, Jenn cooks breakfast and Sharon answers patients' call bells. "Sharon doesn't like cooking that much," says Jenn. Next comes patient care—a bed bath, a shower, mouth care. Jenn asks patients—if they're alert and oriented—what they'd like. "The whole point of people being here," says Jenn, "is keeping them as independent as possible," meaning, for instance, that no one has to wear incontinence briefs—as they might have to do in a nursing home—unless they're actually incontinent.

Since she's been at the Fisher Home, Jenn has learned important lessons about the power of human touch. "I'm not usually much of a hugger," she says, but she finds that just putting her arm around someone or holding a hand can provide emotional support. "I'd want someone to do that for me," she says.

In addition to her floor duties, Jenn has responsibilities as team leader. She has to see that all the documentation is done. Every aide keeps a checklist of the day's shift for each patient: bathing, feeding, toileting. Did she get out of bed? What kind of food did he eat? How much? Were there physical, emotional changes? When the people on the next shift arrive, this documentation helps them know what to expect. Jenn is also responsible for preliminary interviewing and subsequent training of new aides as well as for scheduling all the shifts. New aides shadow a working aide, and spend time finding out what it feels like to be a patient. "We put them into a Hoyer lift to give them that experience, for instance," says Jenn.

The scheduling part of her job is tough, both strategically and emotionally, she says. When she assigns people to shifts, she has to be sure the full-time staff get their choices first; and she needs to consider their seniority at the hospice. "It's hard when you have to call someone and say, 'Sorry, I can't fit you in,' especially when you know they're the only ones working in the family."

Along with one of the nurses, Jenn has been responsible for planning aides' in-service programs, twelve of which are needed each year to keep their licenses. They have had programs on preventing abuse and neglect, on fire safety, on positioning and body mechanics.

How would she like to die? Quickly, in her sleep, and live to be a hundred, as long as she still has a mind. Her daughter has completed her nurse's training, and would be Jenn's advocate. "I wouldn't want to be in pain, and I hope she'd see to it that I wouldn't be, the way I do for people here."

C. died at 1 a.m.; gave body to medical school, but company that trans-
ports wasn't here on time. There is a
strict time limit after death, usually
just a few hours, after which the medical school will not accept it. Gray
SUV eventually arrives, no label on
side, brings gurney covered in dark
green velvet to transport.

Social worker Priscilla relieved
that C.'s situation is resolved--family
very litigious; planning to sue funeral
home, but pleased with Fisher Home.

***

There's a gate across M.'s door--her
cat on the windowsill.

Listened to aide give her report at
the end of her shift. Who had eaten,
how much, who had gotten up to go to
the bathroom, who had had a bowel
movement, how much and what kind: was
it formed? a good amount?

Priscilla says that a new patient has
asked that his second wife not come to
visit, though she wants to. Priscilla
has said she'd speak to the woman.
Sounds like an unpleasant task, but I'm
sure it's not a first for Priscilla.

***

Busy day on Saturday. Seven residents,
another brought in during my stay--
almost a full house. Two nurses--one a
per diem and Matt, a new nurse, plus
two aides, both per diems, so no
really experienced people, no adminis-
trators--and a weekend, so it's hard
to reach doctors. The husband of a new
patient has been staying the nights.
He has dementia and wandered off yesterday. The nice per diem nurse got
into her car and went out looking for
him. They called Ilsa and she came
over to help. The couple's daughter
was in the hospice but not at all
cooperative, not ready to take responsibility for her dad. He's a distin-
guished-looking tall white-bearded
guy, very plausible until you talk to
him. Daughter surly. Some friends
arrive and I show them where the room
is. Husband shows up and they ask him
where his wife is. Oh, she's at home,
he says. No, I say, she's in room 3.
How will this get worked out? Fisher
Home doesn't have the capacity to take
responsibility for a demented spouse
in residence.

A long chat with two other visitors

with questions about insurance and
other matters. I say the social worker
can answer their questions. Also some
concern about medication. Talk to the
clinical staff, I say.

*　*　*

Ilsa shows a film to volunteers, "A
Family Undertaking: Taking Ownership
of Your or Your Loved One's Death and
Burial," a PBS documentary about people keeping their loved ones at home
during the dying process, even burying
them themselves. Parts of it quite
moving--a middle-aged son overcome
with grief, even after much advance
preparation, including having his
father help prepare his own casket;
a reluctant husband whose wife has
insisted on this form of postmortem
wake and burial. Scary, overdone view
of the funeral industry, description
of embalming process--bodies are "bled
and pickled."

Analogies again between birth and
death and the importance of planning
for both, respecting the natural
event, encountering the threshold
between realms. As with natural childbirth, perhaps the same danger here of

fetishizing how it's done, making people
feel guilty about their choices. I
asked if anyone has taken a body home
from the Fisher Home? Answer: no.

A talk with volunteer Joan Roach,
who is part of a group called Sacred
Passage, a free service that helps
families care for loved ones at home
at the time of death and after. Joan
is a retired RN, a follower of the
teachings of Rudolf Steiner, founder
of anthroposophy and the Waldorf
Schools. Steiner, says Joan, teaches
that the soul stays with the body for
three days after death, and that it
remembers the past. The process of
staying with the body helps both dead
and living disconnect, something that
happens too fast in a hospital, she
says, where the body is whisked away.
The group helps with washing and preparing the body for a home vigil and
funeral.

***

Gerard is back from the assisted living place where he was sent, now in
much worse shape. Lucy tells me that
he's aphasic--having trouble speaking--
and experiencing multiple seizures.

When I go in I notice that he seems
unable to use his right hand, but the
eyes are still there. He can do "OK"
and "no," but his mumbled utterances
are not intelligible to me. He no longer has his "M*A*S*H" collection. When
I come in and greet him and reintro-
duce myself, saying I am glad to see
him, he seems pleased. The TV has a
bowling tournament on. Does he want to
watch that? No, he says. When we
finally locate the right remote, I fail
to find something that pleases him. I
then try reading aloud from a poetry
anthology in the room--Frost's "Directive," which probably isn't the right
poem, or maybe none would be. Ask him
if he'd like something to drink. OK.
Some juice? OK. When I bring it in and
present him with a straw to drink it,
he holds it in his mouth, then turns
his head to one side and begins to
tremble. Is this a seizure? I get Lucy,
who attends to him. Lucy thanks me for
letting her know what was happening.
Probably the beginning of a seizure,
but he is having so many of them that
they are hard to keep track of.

I., who has dementia, has been living
at home, and they're seeing if she'll
be able to get used to a new place.
For now she has aides with her most
of the day. The aide today looked
familiar--turned out to be K., who,
after I told her my name, said, "I
took care of your mother." Indeed she
had. She is the one, when I asked her
what to do when Mother asked me if she
was dying, who said she always told
the truth. I had followed her advice,
and Mother had seemed very relieved.

Spend some time helping volunteer
Mary Ann Walker bring in and shelve
the groceries. She is a nutritionist--
by trade, but not official to Fisher
Home--who comes in on Wednesdays to do
some cooking, often some kind of fish.

Sit with a sixty-year-old woman
dying of advanced breast cancer. She
is unresponsive, breathing hard with
occasional groans, but not evidently
in any pain. Completely bald from the
chemo, her skin as smooth as a baby's
and her arms and upper chest look full
and healthy.

Long conversation with new person,
D., who has long-term multiple

sclerosis and some confusion. She is
ambulatory and chatty, though complains that she gets tired out from
friends wanting to talk. Told me she'd
heard that I "do flowers" and asked me
to clean up some of the cut flowers in
her room. She worked at the Survival
Center, had been homeless at one time,
missing teeth in front but otherwise
well groomed and dressed, with longish
gray-blond hair. Tells me that her
daughter has rescheduled her wedding
for a few weeks from now and moved it
to Amherst--evidently with her mother's
condition in mind. D.'s room filled with
Catholic items, little statuette of the
Virgin, Thomas Merton book.

T. has been sleeping in a chair in
the dining room. She wakes up around
lunchtime. Beth Bachand, the aide, has
fixed some attractive small plates with
avocado and tomato. T. would like one.
Ranch dressing is OK. Anything else?
She doesn't like to specify, so I
guess and toast some whole-wheat
bread, butter it, then slice some
pretty good cheddar alongside. Water
with a little ice. There are now lists
on the fridge of people's food likes
and dislikes. Very helpful.

***

The house is full. Lucy Fandel busy
but cheerful, always friendly when I
arrive. How're you doing? I ask, and
she replies, Better since I've seen
you. So that starts things off well
for me. Several new patients, none of
whom I get to meet. They are sleeping--
comatose?--or busy with visitors. The
son-in-law of one new resident is in
the kitchen making tea for himself and
others. Knows how to do this. Asks for
teapot. Aide shows him teakettle. I
look, but don't find a china teapot. He
is pleasant, steeps the tea in mugs.
He is Canadian, down from Ontario. No
wonder he knows tea.

E.'s wife is in a flurry, moving and
talking fast, anxiously. Bringing tray
to kitchen, washing dishes. I tell her
she doesn't need to, but she wants to
keep busy. Understandable. Would she
like to take a break, a walk, a nap,
let me sit with him? No, she's clear
that only she can do this.

Sit with Gerard for a while, watching various sports. I learn that he
once taught phys ed in Grenada, where
he was also getting a medical degree.
Likes soccer, track and field, not

tennis. Too bad for me, because the
U.S. Open is on. He is more articulate
recently, more understandable. Too
bad, again, since his life is so limited. He has had this brain tumor for
more than twelve years.

***

A wedding and three deaths since my
last visit. Norma ecstatic about the
wedding of D.'s daughter--hospice at
its improvisatory best. Several volunteers helped decorate, and Norma and
others made the food, the cake. Wedding
was on Friday, and D. died today, two
days later. She is just being ushered
into the Douglass Funeral Home van on
a red-velvet-covered gurney. When I
accompany T. to the gazebo, we find the
remains of the wedding display, white
tulle ribbons on the floor along with
paper petals, little bouquets of silk
flowers tied with tulle ribbons.

***

I discover that Gerard enjoys the
Sherlock Holmes stories, so I bring in
my childhood volume and am reading the
short ones to him. He has few words,

but has an astonishing recall for the
stories. "Wait," he says, and then
thinks. "It has to do with a stable
nearby." And it turns out a few sen-
tences later that the murderer is hiding
in the stable. Something similar happens
over and over, with different stories,
quite uncanny. When did he last read
these stories? I ask. About forty years
ago. Today he is sleepy and not very
communicative, though sweet and agreeable. Bill Warren, a charming young volunteer, tells me they've put Gerard on
more Ativan lately, which is making him
"loopy." I read "A Scandal in Bohemia,"
using my best German accent to depict
the king. Gerard appears to enjoy that.
I mention his fogginess to Lucy afterward, who says maybe they need to pull
back on the medication.

I sit outside with T., who has Parkinson's and has just been "decertified"--
she's not dying fast enough. She has
been hoping to go home with some live-in
help, but the person backed out at the
last minute. She is very sad. We sit in
the sun and enjoy the falling leaves and
do not talk about her situation. Later I
see aide Beth Bachand sitting with her
on a settee in the hall, talking inti-
mately. I'm sure Beth was a help.

***

A conversation with Priscilla, always
interesting. I tell her I'm going to
the hospital to see a PBS film,
"Consider the Conversation," about
the discussion needed for advance
planning, for clarifying thoughts
about dying, death, and after. She
agrees that it is a hard conversation,
especially for some. Also how to
"sell" hospice--not present it as
hopeless, but hopeful. Some of the
writing promoting it has a syrupy
cast--how to avoid that but give the
real story of what happens.

We talk about the physician-
assisted suicide item on the Massachusetts ballot, the so-called Death With
Dignity initiative. She is for it, as
am I. As with abortion rights, I think
people should be able to choose what
happens to their bodies. Last night an
interview on "Fresh Air" with Judith
Schwartz from something called Compassion and Choices, which helps people
die faster if they wish. All of this
is so much more in the open lately.
Even so, the initiative is voted down.

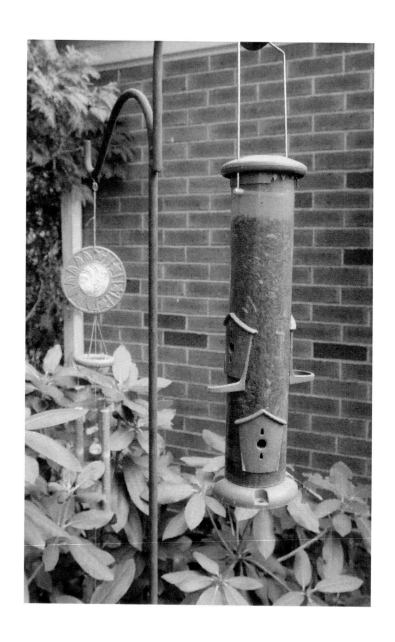

CHAPTER FIFTEEN

FREDERICK GAIGE:
STAYING AT WORK

IN 2001, WHEN FREDERICK GAIGE retired from the presidency of Penn State Berks in Reading, Pennsylvania, at age sixty-four, it was partly because he wanted to do other things. One of those was to try to be a writer. His daughter, novelist Amity Gaige, says that her dad had always had that ambition, but probably had some sort of learning disability. "He was told in sixth grade that he'd never go to college," she says. As it turned out, he not only graduated from college but went on to get his Ph.D., became a college professor and then a highly effective administrator. A specialist in South Asian studies, he had, in fact, already written an admired book on Nepalese politics. But now he wanted to write something else— a fictional account of the distant future. He didn't consider himself a "futurist," although he'd been to a couple of conferences about futurism. "He wanted to be a creative writer," says Amity, but he was a slow at it. He was excited about his project, but soon frustrated when it turned out to be harder than he had expected.

Fred believed strongly that our planet was dying and that it was already too late to save it. He began to think about what would happen to humans, says Amity: "The book was his idea of how we left the planet and what would eventually happen to us as a race—an exciting and ambitious idea." He was always an ambitious person. When he took over the Berks campus, it was a two-year junior college. When he left fifteen years later, he had made it into a four-year residential campus with numerous degree programs and had tripled enrollment. The son, grandson, and great-grandson of college administrators, he was a man with big dreams. "Dad mostly identified himself through his work," his daughter observes, "and through his idealistic and forward-thinking ideas about higher education." Now in retirement, he wanted to try to learn how to do the next thing. He'd gone to a six-week writing program before he got sick. When he arrived at the hospice, he was working hard on his book.

Amity, whose mother is a family therapist, describes both of her parents as "workaholics," with high standards about what they should do and what others should do for the community. It never occurred to her that people would take jobs they didn't care about, since her relationship with her dad involved watching him doing work he loved. But that relationship also involved his unstinting encouragement of her work as a writer, starting when she was seven or eight. "He was a great father," she says.

When Fred arrived at the Fisher Home in the spring of 2009, his daughter was able to return the life-long compliment, and help him with his writing. During the six months until his death on August 25, he would sit in a chair or in his bed and write on lined yellow pads in his large, flowing handwriting. Then she and some of the hospice volunteers would type the pages into his laptop as he read them aloud. He finished the book, although it wasn't as long as it would have been had he survived. Amity had it copied and bound, though she's not necessarily thinking of having it published more widely. "He didn't believe in an afterlife," she says, "so I don't think of him there watching me." Then she qualifies that assessment. "Well, he did believe in the afterlife, in that there was energy going on—reincarnation in a certain sense."

The gist of his book, she says, is that people were "still evolving as human beings, and that we were going to evolve out of our bodies and would become just consciousness, a process that would take many, many years." She believes he melded ideas about evolution with his knowledge of Eastern religions to conclude that we would gain a kind of enlightenment through this evolutionary process.

Here are a few excerpts from Fred Gaige's book, *I Am God*:

> I think of the human exploration of deep space as a vibrant, growing tree, expanding skyward over time to include more and more planetary settlements. . . . Then around one billion years post-Earth-2 settlements, two major breakthroughs occurred. Scientists discovered how to travel instantaneously from one planetary settlement to the next. . . .
>
> Project managers fretted over the selection of settlers, worried that the frontier mentality of those

attracted to this adventure was the same loner arche-
type of those who, at least in popular lore, conquered
the West with guns in hand.

Then, many eons into the future, evolutionary changes
happen, and the first-person narrator comes into being.

The Caliban and Canali people evolved physically into
pieces of their mother star, round glowing heads and
just enough arm and leg appendages to manipulate the
machinery of their everyday responsibilities. . . . [They]
began to experience the appearance on the scene of
many seers. One of them was me. Over thousands
of years I meditated and was honored by the people of
Canali for the power of my connectedness to God.

Fred was happy at the Fisher Home, says Amity.
Although he had bladder cancer that had moved into
his liver and then bones, for the first three months it
almost seemed as if he were well. Amity was happy
with her experience there, too. "I have really fond
memories of it. Funny, considering that time of my life
was so intense." She was teaching creative writing at
Amherst College, had a three-and-a-half-year-old son,

and was working on a novel, which became the much-praised *Schroder*. She would work at the library in the morning, go and see her dad at the hospice, then pick up her son at day care. She was, she says, "in the process of losing my mind." Because her parents had separated shortly before Fred got sick, his care had fallen to her. "In the normal situation, it would have been my mom taking care of him," she says. Her mother was, in fact, a regular visitor, and it seems that her parents worked things out in those last months. "How wonderful," says Amity, "to have a period of time when you can make peace with somebody, know that death is coming, instead of doing all of this waiting and putting off because you think there's one more solution and one more thing to be tried."

She learned at the hospice that dying doesn't happen overnight—"if it's done right." She came to understand that "a patient in hospice participates in his own death in a way that somebody that's under medical intervention really doesn't." She believes that medical intervention is sometimes just denial, and it prevents the "beautiful emotional transformation" that she saw her father go through. Because Fred came to the hospice before he was too terribly ill, she believes it was the right path for them. In addition, she thinks that her father had "an amazing ability to accept the fact of his dying and to use his time, not sit there and mope or look out the window. He wanted to continue to work, which is what he loved to do, and that was completely acceptable." In addition, she felt that anything she wanted to do at the Fisher Home was okay: "I even brought him a couple of beers once when he was having a craving. It was exactly what he needed and wanted." She thinks the great sin would be to deny a dying person what he wants. The dying person gets to make the choice.

Still, she says, "It's amazing how negatively people react to death. There's a close friend, a person I've always admired, who was so angry at Fred for deciding to go into hospice that he refused to see him until he reconsidered chemotherapy. I was thinking: 'What are you implying? That he doesn't want to live? That he hasn't tried hard enough? That he should be suffering more?' The friend finally came around and came to the hospice, and they did things together and he was helpful in the end." There are people, she says, "who can't tolerate the fact that someone is dying—so they just want to do something about it. But that's about them, not about the dying person." Amity understands that it's often families who don't want dying people to enter hospice care, and she's proud of the fact that she didn't try to talk her father out of it. "When I found him, he was in a rehab center in Brooklyn, sharing a room with some guy on his last legs, with the TV blaring and trucks going by. This is where somebody wants to stay, and then maybe get more chemo and then maybe die there? No."

At the Fisher Home, she says, he had what seemed to her the best room—sunny, at the end of the hall. He had his own bathroom. "He had all the care he needed, and it was beautiful. I always liked going there. It was the most transcendent thing I've ever done, besides childbirth—being with my dad for that period of time. I felt really lucky to have had that time with him, and really glad for him that he had this gift, which was acceptance. He lived a long life; he got to do some of the things he really wanted to do. One last thing he had to do was write a book, so that's what he did.

"If you look at the bright side of terminal illness, there's this opportunity to have everybody let go of the person, including the person himself let go of himself. And it's a long process. It's hard to let go of yourself, hard to let go of life. It took him a long time to let go.

But how wonderful to have that opportunity, like giving birth—so you're pregnant for nine months; the baby grows really big to the point where you just want the baby out of you. Then the baby's born. That's the way our psychology handles things. We need nine months to be born, and maybe nine months to die— it would be symmetrical that way. Psychologically, spiritually—probably we have to occur to ourselves and then forget ourselves. He did that, I saw him let go of layers one by one. It was amazing to see. There was the recognizable Fred—the daily self, then the self who's a patient, a sick person; then that layer gets shed, and that's really the end. Even in the hallucinating, they're in a different world altogether—they're not even in hospice anymore. They're already gone. They're going somewhere. They see it."

After Fred got really sick, the doctor in New York told him that if he went through chemo again, it might kill him. At that point Amity didn't know anything about the Fisher Home. She was in an airport, in the bar. "I don't like to fly, so I have a drink before I get on the plane, and a woman came and sat down next to me, and after I told her where I was from, she said, 'Oh, Amherst, that's where my mother-in-law is in hospice care.' I asked her more about it, and she said, there's this wonderful place—and that's how I found it. And then I went to see Dad and said, you know, I just heard about this hospice." She never got the woman's name. "She was a guardian angel. I don't even know if she was real."

Hurricane Sandy is arriving sometime
today. I have been for a walk down to
the Grist Mill and back, only a few
cars still on the road. Colleges
closed, state offices. I call Ilsa to
say I will not be coming in today, per
the official advice, though at the
moment nothing is happening except
anticipation and a little wind and
some mistiness.

***

Read "The Red-headed League" to
Gerard. He enjoys as always, as do I.
I ask him how he is doing. He pauses,
then replies: "Next question." When I
leave, he asks when am I coming back.
He is sadder than usual today. Priscilla tells me that he knows they will
need evidence that he's declining,
because otherwise they might have to
decertify him and move him out again.
Awful. These are the Medicare rules,
alas. I tell Ilsa I feel bad not to
spend more time with Gerard. She
reminds me that volunteers should try
not to get too attached to residents.
I am aware of this, but feel bad all
the same. I know that this is also a
problem for staff at times. Some

people just connect with you more than
others. Volunteers and staff need to
mourn, too, at times.

***

It's November 2012. We're told that a
new director has been appointed.

***

A fascinating encounter with K., a
woman with Lewy body syndrome. Another
woman in the house has it, too. Its
victims show a bipolar type of behavior, alternating agitation and energy
with extreme lethargy. K.'s daughter
tells me that her mother had once
played the trombone, been an avid
skier, in general had been a lively
and engaged person.
    K. lies in her bed, tangled in the
sheets, moving restlessly, wide awake.
I straighten out her covers a bit,
then ask about playing the trombone.
"Oh, no, she says," I never played the
trombone." I don't disagree. Then
after a while she says, "I falsified
the documents." "Oh," I ask, "what
documents?" And she says, "The ones
about playing the trombone. I really

can't play it." Never mind, I say, and
ask if she'd like a little back rub.
I gently rub her back, shoulder, and
arm, which she seems to like, then
sing a little: "Loch Lomond," "Danny
Boy," and some Christmas carols. After
a while she says, "Don't sing." So I
stop, but continue to rub her back.
Then a little later, she says, "Sing
some more," so I do. "I can't sing,"
she says, and then, "I'm a deaf mute."
I ask her if she likes having me rub
her back, and she says yes, but then,
"Don't you get sick of doing that?"
No, I say, I rather enjoy it. Lucy
comes in and administers some meds in
chocolate ice cream. Eventually K.
turns onto her other side. I ask if
she'd like to go to sleep. She says
yes, and I leave.

Staff and volunteers have our
annual "Jeopardy"-type game, run by
one of the nurses, to go over the
federal OSHA and HIPAA regulations.
These deal with safety, protection
from infection, and privacy. All volunteers have to pass an annual review
of these, as do staff. The nurse has
invented a quiz-show format that makes
this serious subject a lot more fun.
We gather--some twenty of us--in the

living room and divide up into teams.
Of course the team with the most
nurses has the biggest advantage, but
it is a time for both congeniality and
education. We answer, among others,
questions about transmission of the
various forms of hepatitis; the best
way to avoid transmission of infec-
tions. Answer: frequent hand washing.

***

We've learned that the new director,
Maxine Stein, will be coming to work
in a couple of weeks. So far, everyone
who has met or known her is full of
enthusiasm. There will be changes,
surely, the first of which is to find
office space for her. Evidently an
architect is at work on this and other
physical changes. It has been over a
year since Greg left, and things have
been fraying around the edges.

I arrive to a slippery parking lot
and offer to put down some sand. Lucy
says: Help me out with this first. M.'s
mother, who lives in Boston, is on the
phone, wanting to say some words to
her daughter. M. is in her sixties.
Mother has not wanted to see her
daughter in the hospital or hospice,

because she wants to remember her as
healthy and beautiful. M. is now
skeletal--cancer of some sort--only
one eye really opens, teeth too big
for her mouth, in the way of shrinking
bodies. She lies mostly on her right
side with arms folded and crossed on
her chest, more or less fetal position. Occasionally she says a few
words, but mostly the sounds she makes
are not decipherable. I am to pick up
the phone when Lucy transfers the call
and put it to M.'s left ear. I do this
and try to see whether she is responding. She blinks a bit, as usual, but
it's hard to see much else in the way
of response. I can't hear what the
mother is saying, but when I hear
beeping from the phone, I know the
call is over.

Lucy comes in and asks M. if she's
heard what her mother said. M. gives
a slight nod. "She is with you in
spirit," says Lucy.

I stay for a while, holding M.'s
hands, lightly rubbing her arms and
almost hairless head. I sing a few old
songs, "Loch Lomond," "Auld Lang Syne"
for New Year's. She makes a few
responsive nods and grunts, then tries
hard to say something--umm, umm. I try

to suggest what that might be--Mother?
After a while she begins to seem quite
restless. I ask her if she's in pain.
No response. Then I ask, "Do you
hurt?" "All over," she says quite
clearly. I go to find Lucy and some
medical help.

In the living room a more cheerful
scene is unfolding. Y., a longtime
Amherst resident I know by sight, is
now living here. Her daughter, with
whom she's been living for the past
few years, is making a cell-phone call
in the dining room. Her granddaughters
and the family dog are entertaining Y.
I sit on the floor and play with the
cute dog, a rescue animal, small,
lively, and willing to give me her
paws in rapid succession. One of the
granddaughters is living in Portland,
Oregon, where our youngest son lives,
and we exchange observations about the
city. She is hoping to move back east.

I go out to the parking lot with
some sand, where George Maston is
energetically shoveling parking spaces
the plow has missed. This has not been
well taken care of in previous years,
but it's the sort of thing a new
director should be able to take in
hand. Let's hope.

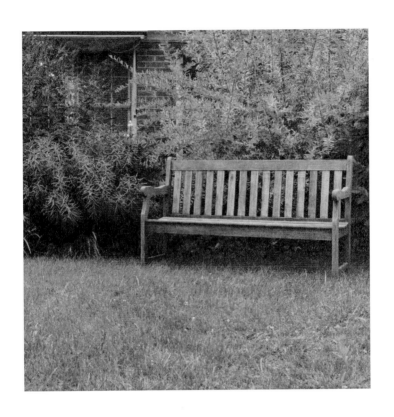

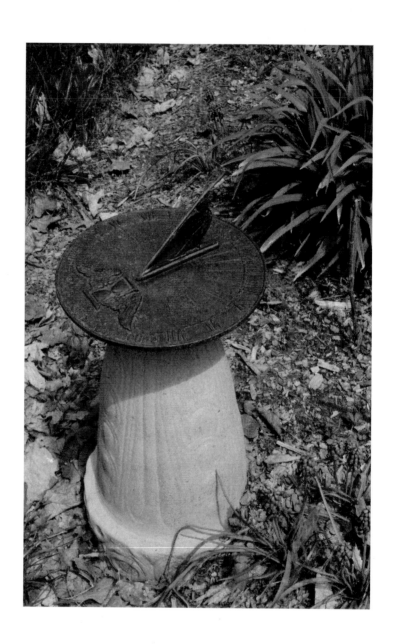

CHAPTER SIXTEEN

VOLUNTEERS:

A RANGE OF EXPERIENCE

The Kellys: Finding Meaning in Retirement

MANY HOSPICE VOLUNTEERS come to the Fisher Home after experiencing the death of a significant person in their lives. Some are young, but most are older people with the benefit or burden of considerable life experience. A few, like Bob and Janine Kelly, come as couples. Both Kellys are retired teachers in town; Bob taught high school social studies, and Janine was an elementary school special education teacher. They live more or less around the corner from the Fisher Home, and their retirements coincided closely with the opening of the hospice. Both were clear that after retirement, they didn't want to "just sit around."

They became volunteers at Grace Episcopal Church, where Janine worked with a group that provided companionship to elderly people. Bob joined the vestry, sang in the choir, and helped out with fund-raising. When Janine's mother was nearing the end of her life, they had discussed the possibility of bringing her up from Connecticut to the newly established hospice, but the eighty-three-year-old lady adamantly wanted to remain at home. At the end, she had hospice care there, but only for a short time. "They were wonderful," says Janine, and it made her and Bob think they'd like to get involved in something similar.

Bob's retirement was more gradual than some. He had decided to do part-time work after 2004, and then took a medical leave after he was diagnosed with leukemia, from which he is now fully recovered. He returned to teach part-time before finally leaving the school in 2007.

The day Janine retired, her colleagues took her out to a restaurant next door to the Hospice Shop. She stopped in just to find out what it was like. They wanted her to start volunteering right away, so she did, and eventually became interim manager of the shop. Bob joined in as a gofer: "I drive stuff back and forth."

At the Fisher Home the Kellys have often worked outdoors as gardeners, weeding, raking, and planting, but most of their volunteer time is spent indoors with residents. That's the real pleasure, says Bob—"You meet some very interesting people at a special stage of life." He had already spent quite a bit of time thinking about this subject. At the high school, he created a course on death and dying, comparing theories and writings with people's realities. At the Fisher Home, he deals with the realities. "People arrive here in very different places emotionally. Some stay in that place, and some change. Some are open, some closed." The critical role of the volunteer, Bob thinks, is not to try to talk about ultimate things unless the person is open to that, but rather to discover what the person is interested in. He's learned a lot from people—from one, for instance, who was a descendant of several generations of Amherst residents, about the history of the town.

Says Janine, "I think one of the pluses to be with people at that point in their life is that they don't have any pretenses—very different from the working world." So you learn to be open to wherever a person is on a given day. "That's a gift that you're getting. I think we almost get more than we give at times."

Right, says Bob. "And I think it's important not to think too hard that we're giving a gift: 'This is what I'm going to do for you, whether you want it or not.'" He sees that as a misunderstanding of the volunteer's role. "A lot of us who go into that type of work, whether as volunteers or as careers, do it for somewhat selfish reasons," and in hospice work, even for the paid staff, it can't be for the money. "But whether we're looking for something to enhance our lives, fill in something that's missing—as I used to tell the kids in the classroom, it's not automatically a bad thing. The key is what you do with that, and that you don't exploit people."

Hospice volunteers are taught—and reminded from time to time—that they need to observe boundaries in their relationships with residents, that these relationships need to stay inside the Fisher Home. But even within the hospice, there need to be boundaries. Janine recalls one resident who liked to talk to her about a daughter with whom she had a difficult relationship. "She would say to me, 'Well, what would you do?' And I would usually just turn it back to her and say, 'Have you talked to your daughter about this?' " Professional expertise can produce its boundary problems, too, says Bob. "Let's say one of the volunteers has a medical background, then that person has to remember that it doesn't give you powers and responsibilities higher than or different from the rest of the volunteers. You can go to the on-duty nurse and say, 'Hey, you might want to check this out,' not, 'You should be doing . . .' " On the other hand, Janine has found that the nursing staff is very receptive when she tells them that something seems strange or different with a resident. They'll go right in and check on the person.

Both Kellys have high praise for the staff. "They're compassionate and like what they're doing," says Janine. But they see a difference in attitude when the regular staff is replaced by per diem hires. Yet even the seasoned regulars will occasionally clash with a resident. "Yes," says Bob, "some patients are very difficult. We volunteers can avoid them; the staff can't." He remembers one resident who cursed at people, one who exploded into violence just before dying. But, says

Bob, training is crucial. "If you can't deal with it, then you've got to seek another line of work."

Training is crucial for volunteers, too, they agree, but add that much of the learning happens on the job at the Fisher Home. Janine thinks the times when volunteers get together for discussion or to watch a film or hear a talk are also extremely valuable, since volunteers rarely see each other otherwise. Volunteer coordinator Ilsa Myers organizes these in-service events. "In the meeting format," says Janine, "that's where you get to share what you've learned, talk about problems."

One thing both of them have learned is that they wouldn't mind ending up here. "Absolutely," says Bob.

Deb Gorlin: Observing the Process

DEB GORLIN MINCES FEW WORDS. "I got interested in volunteering for hospice for a number of reasons," she explains, "not many of them selfless." A poet and a teacher of creative writing at Hampshire College, she is also a breast cancer survivor: "I got interested in hospice because I'm curious about dying, and I wanted to see the process, the passage, up front, close, and personal. I wasn't satisfied by anyone else's descriptions, and there weren't that many that strike me as palpable and tangible." There was also, she says, a desire to help people at that stage, in part having to do with her inability to do that when her own parents died. Her father dropped dead in the shower at age sixty-five, when she was twenty-eight. Fifteen years later, her mother had one of her numerous episodes of congestive heart failure while living in a nursing home in Florida. She was sent to the hospital in an ambulance and died on the way. And Deb remembers thinking: "Well, there must be better ways of dying than that."

When a good friend was dying of cancer, Deb and another friend nursed her and were present at her death. Deb found the experience fascinating, moving, and disturbing: "I felt that I wanted practice, some experiences I could draw from, some resources on how to die that I could draw upon when my time came, when my loved ones' times came. It was a way to integrate it into my life experience so that I could address and be competent about it." It's a really interesting subject, she says. "I joke about myself being a kind of experience slut."

She doesn't see herself as a Good Samaritan—"'Aren't I a good girl, ministering to the ill and the dying.' When people say, 'Oh, you're so brave,' I don't take that seriously." She compares herself to a surgeon, able to dissociate herself from the experience and not be overwhelmed by it. It's much easier, of course, because these are for the most part people she does not have close relationships with. It was different with her friend. "I certainly felt the grief and pain there."

One thing she worries about with hospice is that the experience of working with the dying could become numbing, "so 'normalized' that I don't recognize it in the here and now because my mind is elsewhere. So if doing this kind of work is spiritual—and I put 'spiritual' in big quotation marks—then what I am doing is trying to stay in this experience so that it stays meaningful, and not let it get overlaid or distracted by all the other concerns in my life. That's another reason I do it, is that it is in some ways a total escape from my everyday life and complaints and aggravations." It's only human to get habituated, so we have to keep reminding ourselves, she says, "Hey, wait a minute: death down the hall."

Volunteering can be full of surprises. A resident's

daughter asked Deb to keep her dad company while the daughter went out for a while. The man told her about his life as an engineer, how he'd had two ex-wives and a girlfriend. Then he told Deb he'd seen her on eHarmony, an online dating site. "He said, 'You fit the description: striking, gray hair, writer.' And I said to myself, 'You can't be hitting on me!' " She told him he was mistaken, unless she had a double somewhere. "I was thinking, 'Well, wait a minute, you have a girlfriend. What are you doing?' It was an odd moment."

She sees that moment as in some ways defining the difference between a volunteer's and a staffer's relationship with residents. She has seen aides gently but firmly correcting behavior, drawing the line. She describes a scene in which one elderly woman with slight dementia was sitting at the dining room table with other residents and loudly informed an aide: "You have big tits." The aide, normally a good-humored woman, turned to the resident and said, "Am I correct in hearing what you just said?" The resident then turned to another resident and said, "And you're ugly." At that point, says Deb, the aide took the woman's wheelchair and scooted her out the door and into her room, saying, "I think you need a time-out." Deb admired the aide's response. "They have an intimacy with people, a relationship that involves their bodies. You can't get more intimate than changing people's incontinence briefs," she says. And that intimacy allows them to treat people not as dying patients, but as "people who have to be accountable, who have some agency and an obligation to be kind and not say thoughtless things. It's real."

Volunteers, by contrast, have to maintain a kind of distance, and that's appropriate: "We're there for just a few hours a week, so people's behavior is not going to get under our skin. We're not living with them the way the staff are." In general at the Fisher Home, she sees "a real attempt to get to know who the person is, aside from the dying. I remember being struck the first few weeks that I was there that, Hold on, these people are dying, but—and it sounds kind of crazy—but they're still people." The hospice philosophy works here, she thinks: "If at all possible, I'd like to die at home, but if I can't, then this is about as good as it gets." Death is not pathologized—not treated as if it were a disease—at the Fisher Home, she says. People are comfortable. "Everybody is an individual. It's not a factory farm. A lot of that has to do with the size of the place, and that it is a home. There's a backyard where you can see the birds, where you can sit outside, and your family can come and visit and not have to go down to the gift shop or the snack bar and get food from machines."

Deb feels this is the best volunteer work she can do. She's not good at meetings, she says, not good at canvassing or volunteering for political, ecological, or environmental groups, even the ones she supports. "I don't feel that's my gift, where I'm at ease." For her, hospice is "the perfect cause, because it's one-on-one and has to do with major transitions in life, a major existential passage. The only other comparably meaningful passage would be birth." Working here, she says, has "informed" her. "I can draw from my knowledge with examples of how other people have gone from the world that make up, I think, for the deaths of my parents. When the time comes, I may be able to put that into action."

Bill Warren: Discovering What's Important

AT TWENTY-ONE, Bill Warren is one of the younger volunteers. A junior chemistry major at UMass, he brings to the hospice what volunteer coordinator Ilsa

Myers describes as a breath of fresh air. He comes regularly on the weekends on foot from the campus where he lives, a mile and a half away. Tall, gangly, and somewhat tousle-headed, he has a relaxed manner and an easy laugh, but he is completely serious about volunteering at the Fisher Home. "Student life is so far removed from everything. I came to the hospice to learn what people find important, what they are thinking about at this time of life, to put things into perspective," he says.

He's been a volunteer for a little over a year, and has found it satisfying, even uplifting. He was surprised at first to find the atmosphere so upbeat, and has been pleased to have a chance to learn about people's lives, both from the residents and from their families. The volunteer training got him thinking about questions he otherwise wouldn't have asked himself, questions about the end of life: Would you want to be kept alive? On a respirator? Have someone feed you? As he puts it: Who thinks about those things when you're twenty-one? He had previously considered burial versus cremation and had come down firmly on the side of cremation, "because of the chemistry," he says. "Everything breaks down into its elements. I like the idea of the energy being given off. It's kind of cool. Then burial at sea. That's the way to go."

The importance of hospice came home strongly to him recently when his grandfather, someone he had been close to, died in a hospice residence at age ninety-one. He had been doing pretty well after being treated for colon cancer, but he had a sudden decline, says Bill, and went to the hospital on a Saturday and then to hospice, where he spent less than a day. Even in that short time, he notes, his parents were very appreciative of the kindness and attention he got at the hospice. "As a hospice volunteer," he says, "you don't realize the effect you have on people—just being there makes a difference."

Bill was brought up Catholic but is "not so much of one anymore." He thinks everyone has a religious side—" 'No atheists in foxholes.' You turn to whatever comforts you in an emergency." He says yes to an afterlife and especially likes the idea of the Native American spirits, the sun, the ocean, a reverence for the idea of life.

He tries to bring what he can to the Fisher Home's residents—conversation, silence, whatever they seem to want. Some people don't want you there at all, and that's okay, too, he says. One of the favorite parts of his regular visit is reading the narrative notes in Ilsa's office, where other volunteers write about their experiences with residents: "You learn about people's bios. Then you can sit with them and appreciate who they are." Humor can be an invaluable asset, he feels. "The right person can brighten someone's day—I don't want to say by distracting them from the inevitable end, but to an extent to get them out of their own head. That's really my goal with some people."

One of the most moving conversations he's had was with Dr. Gerard Sterling. They talked about physician-assisted suicide, the so-called Death With Dignity proposition, which was voted down in Massachusetts in 2012. Gerard had said that although he didn't necessarily agree with the law, he was in favor of it selfishly, for himself. Of course, even if the law had passed, the lethal medication would not have been provided in a hospice.

Bill recognizes the advantages to being a young volunteer: "When I walk into a room with someone who's a great deal older than me, there's a certain ranking of things. If they are verbal, it's almost as if they're teaching—'This is what I want to tell you, young'un.' Sometimes that's a good dynamic to have, to get people talking. You're a surrogate grandchild, and they can pass on their wisdom."

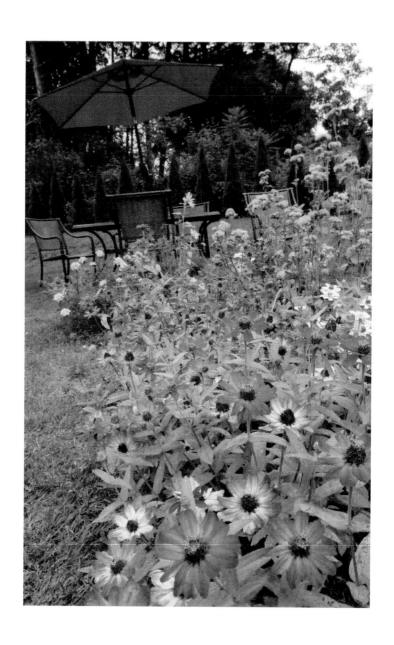

CHAPTER SEVENTEEN

ALI DIAMOND:
THE SHOP,
A CRUCIAL BUTTRESS

ALI DIAMOND HAS BEEN managing the Fisher Home's Hospice Shop since the spring of 2009. The shop, which is the hospice's main fund-raiser, is located in a small strip mall on a direct path between Route 9 and the University of Massachusetts. A popular stopping place for people looking for gently used clothing and small housewares, it's been a huge success. In 2013, its annual Fall Turnover Day broke a record with $7,500 in sales. People had lined up before the shop opened to get at the bargains. The day's take contributed to a total of over $240,000 for the year. This extra money goes to help the hospice serve people who cannot afford its daily rate.

Ali's father ran a used-book store, and she has mostly worked in small independent businesses. As the hospice shop manager, she says, her concerns are the same as for any other retail store: quality control, stocking, merchandising, and promotion. But here, instead of hired staff, she works with volunteers— about sixty of them, and two paid assistant managers. At just thirty, Ali is more like a daughter or grand-daughter to the mostly women volunteers, whose average age is about sixty-five. Two retired men help manage the shop's storage facility and do all sorts of repairs and improvements. "We have a wonderful group of volunteers, very dedicated," Ali says. Still, a lot of that dedication is the result of her efforts, as she puts it, "to make sure people feel appreciated, that they're happy and feeling useful." People also need to work well together. "Slight intuition has gone a long way," she says, in guessing how people's personalities are going to mix when she puts them on the same three-hour shift.

She finds out what people's preferences are and makes her assignments accordingly. "If you don't want to work a cash register, you're not going to work a cash register, ever. If you want to interact with customers, then you'll be on the floor. If you don't want to interact, you can be out back," sorting or steaming wrinkled clothes. The volunteers pick their spots, and then everyone is happier.

Longtime volunteer Libby Klekowski can attest to

the congenial atmosphere. Ali knows how to find the right person for each job, she says; she sets a good tone and she's full of enthusiasm: "She's wanted our customers to feel they're coming to a boutique, not a thrift shop." When she started volunteering in 2008, Libby felt she didn't have the skills to work in the hospice residence, but she wanted to help support its mission. A collaborator with her husband on several books, she has wound up sorting and pricing the many volumes that come into the shop.

The shop is set up with different areas for different items—clothing, linens, housewares, books. Says Ali, "We'll brainstorm ideas for displays, themes in the front room around different holidays, seasonal things"—Christmas gifts, a spring garden table. This is what people see when they walk in. These presentations are accomplished by meticulously managing donations throughout the year, setting aside items for particular displays. Space is always a challenge because when the shop is open for business, it's also open for donations. The donation area, almost as big as the sales area, is where clothing and other items are sorted. Items the shop can't use are passed along to the Salvation Army or the Amherst Survival Center. "The Salvation Army comes several times a week to do pickups. They're able to take things we can't sell, with a stain or a hole." They do a business in rags, and can recycle textiles—things that are torn or have no buttons. Often the shop sends the Survival Center items that simply haven't sold or things that come in big quantities— "twenty pairs of men's pants that come in at the same time."

Turnover is the name of the game in this shop, so for regular customers, there's always something new to look at. Ali prices goods with a color tag. "For a two-week period, we'll use blue. Then after two weeks we'll switch to another color. Then there'll be a week in between and the blue will go on sale." The sale is half price, and the stock is controlled without the staff having to go out on the floor and pull things all the time. The only time that system doesn't apply is the period right after the spring and fall turnovers, when everything is new. Before the turnovers, the shop closes for one day and everything in the store is cleared out. About a dozen volunteers come in and remove all the clothing destined for the Survival Center or local shelters, depending on what they need. The group vacuums the whole place, polishes all the racks, then restocks. "We really go crazy," says Ali, "and it's a lot of fun."

Aide Beth Bachand tells me about her
views of the afterlife. Well, not
exactly, but after her brother died--
here at the Fisher Home--she was out
driving and a hawk suddenly swooped
down on her car. Same thing happened
to her brother's wife. Was he sending
a message--Don't lose sight of me? In
the recent French film "Amour," about
an elderly couple facing the wife's
decline and death, there are a touching
few moments with a pigeon that gets
into the house by mistake, is let out,
then is captured on its second entry.

***

A cautionary tale: An elderly gent
with serious heart problems had the
habit of keeping his Do Not Resuscitate papers in his pocket when he went
out for a morning walk. He collapsed
by the side of the road, and the ambulance EMTs did not look for or find
those orders. They rushed him to the
hospital and revived him. He was furious. When he arrived at the Fisher
Home, he told the nurses and others
that he wanted to die. He was still
walking and talking clearly, but died
two days later.

***

Maxine Stein has made a big difference
already, mostly physical. Rearranging,
creating new offices, new spaces, with
quite a bit of carpentry and flurry.
There is an air of expectancy and
invigoration.

Meanwhile, Gerard is going down-
hill, but so slowly that it is painful
for everyone. Ilsa passed along word
that we're not to feed him except at
mealtimes--not "recreationally," that
is. I had earlier made him an ice
cream, banana, and orange juice
smoothie with Sharon, the aide's,
blessing. I had to feed him with a
spoon. He doesn't have words--though
he echoed my "Bye-bye"--but the personality is still there.

Moving conversation with the daughter
of a new resident. Mother independent
until the dog died, then had a heart
attack, followed by stroke. Now dying,
but family all gathering round, including a nephew who is here with his fiddle
to play for her. As T., the daughter,
weeps, I find myself in tears as well.
She turns out to be a classmate of one
of our sons at Amherst High, class of
'79. Beth, the aide is, too.

***

Lucy asks me to look in on Q. She is
over ninety, a former prof of Spanish
and Portuguese at UMass, a distinguished scholar. She has been crying
out. I introduce myself and sit with
her. Try talking, but she is incoher-
ent, hard to understand. A few things--
"apple juice, hello, no"--but other
speech is garbled. I try reading from
the Renaissance Center's newsletter,
which I find on her windowsill. Not
much interest. Try singing--she asks
me to be quiet. But when I show her
the flowers from her windowsill--tulips
and daffodils--she brightens and says,
"lovely." But she cannot find a comfortable place to settle, her big,
knotted hands working away at the covers, her deep-socketed eyes opening
and closing with an expression of
worry and puzzlement. She seems to be
trying to sit up, so I raise the bed
a bit. Doesn't help. Stroking her arm
and forehead seem to make her more
anxious. But the flowers evidently give
her some pleasure.

In another room a daughter is trying to persuade her mother, I., that
she is in the right place. The mother

has rectal cancer, and they have
stopped treating it, but the mother
is not ready to accept that, thinks
more could be done. The conversation
is conducted at high volume and with
the door open. I'm uncomfortable and
mention this to Lucy. She says, well,
they have to work this out. She's
right.

In Room 4, Gerard's bed has been
moved to the opposite wall, and he is
sleeping flat on his back, very serene.
He does not respond to the sound of my
voice. He looks quite young.

***

Saturday's visit produces some interesting contrasts. I encounter L. in
the dining room, a spiky woman who's
lived in her own house until now. She
has finished her breakfast and is
sitting there alone, with her usual
sour expression, the Gazette, the
Northampton paper, on the table near
her. I know she wants the Springfield
paper and ask if it has come yet. No,
and she is disgusted. How is she today?
I ask--knowing it's a dangerous question. "Alive," she says, "damn it!"
A retired nurse, she has end-stage

cancer and is not, so far as I know,
in pain but no longer able to live in
her own house, where her son had been
taking care of her. Last week, I
played bingo with L., her son, and
another daughter. She has five attentive children, to whom she complains
constantly about being here. It is a
beautiful day, and I ask if she'd like
to go out. She shrugs, makes a face
and says, "Whatever." I take her out
into the sun, walk around the grounds
a bit, and look at the early crocuses
and other bulbs coming up through the
scruffy remains of winter. I spot one
yellow crocus by the driveway that is
blooming all alone. "Look," I say. And
she sees it and actually says "Nice."
     We go back to the main door and
plant ourselves in the sun, listening
to the crows make a racket overhead.
We don't talk much after I've asked
her whether she's had a garden. "Of
course," she says. What did she grow?
"Everything--flowers, vegetables, some
lilacs." And, she adds, "They should
let you stay in your own house!" I see
her point. So we sit in the sun, and
after a while I say, "The sun is nice,
isn't it?" She agrees.
     I visit Q. again. A lot of the time

she is calling out "Hello, hello!" in
a loud voice. I now know not to talk
too much or to sing. She has made that
clear. But the last time I was with
her I showed her the flowers on her
windowsill, and that seemed to please
her. I try the same today, with the
same result. When I put the flowers
away and sit down next to her, she
reaches out toward me. I am wearing a
brightly colored scarf that gets her
attention. I take it off and give it
to her to touch and look at. She makes
happy sounds. So for Q., pleasure is
visual, color and pattern.

***

Gerard died early this morning. I was
there yesterday by his bedside, singing and stroking his shoulder while he
breathed intermittently but steadily.
He had an odd smell, something he'd
had in the past week or so. Beth said
they hadn't been brushing his teeth,
but the smell was coming from deeper
inside. I'd smelled it with Sara, too.
He already looked dead, his skin gray
and his cheeks sunken. Priscilla
stopped in and said she thought his
spirit had already left and that only

his body was still there. Lucy says he'd
always had the heart of an athlete, a
slow, steady, strong beat. I had sung
some hymns, which may not have been
especially appropriate, since he never
expressed any religious feeling to me.
Still I had "Jesus, Lover of My Soul"
welling up. I didn't sing the words,
only the tune--Aberystwyth, that great
Welsh melody--and "The Ash Grove" and
"Where'er You Walk." Rest in peace,
Gerard.

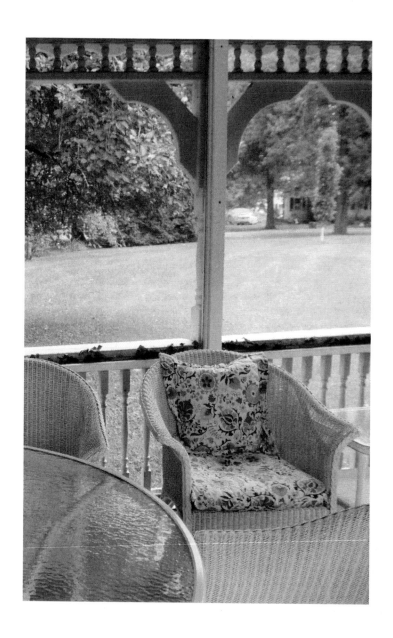

CHAPTER EIGHTEEN

Veterans:
bringing them home

Georges Shally was a strong man, both physically and mentally, always eager to take on new challenges. He had been an executive at Crown Zellerbach, one of the country's biggest paper companies, and his widow, Connie, describes him as an unusual person. "He could do anything he set his mind to"—building houses, sculpting marble, creating gardens, traveling the world at the drop of a hat. He could do all those things, that is, until his mind began to be eaten up by Alzheimer's disease eight years before his death. Connie took care of him first at their home in New Jersey and then for the past five years at home in Amherst. George died on June 25, 2013, at the Fisher Home. He was eighty-seven and had been there a little over six weeks.

George served in the U.S. Army during World War II, in two of that war's toughest places, the Battle of the Bulge, where 19,000 Americans died, and later on the island of Luzon, where he and his division were charged with rounding up Japanese soldiers who were hiding in caves, unaware that the war had ended. What he told his family about those times were mostly amusing escapades, not stories about being scared, not about the shooting and carnage, nor about the deaths of friends or enemies. One from his time on Luzon—where the weather was terrible, hot, rainy and buggy—involves a piano. The Americans were spending a lot of time sitting around in their barracks playing cards, and George found out that one of his buddies played the piano. "If we had music," Connie quotes him as saying, "we wouldn't be so miserable with all this rain." So without asking for official permission, he and his friends simply got in a truck, drove up to the officers' club, and said, "We've come for the piano," then drove off with it.

Charming and agreeable all his life, at the end George became hard to deal with. Still a big man, six feet tall and vigorous, he turned combative, cursed at people, wouldn't let them touch him. When Connie took him to the hospital for an evaluation, she says, he was treated with "heavy antipsychotics" and didn't respond well. So she contacted the Fisher Home, who did their own evaluation and decided to admit him. Gradually, she says, the hospice staff took away the medications a little at a time and were able to build the trust that made him more comfortable. "They treated him like a real person, not just someone they had to tie down, and he gradually got used to being there," says Connie. When the family was there, he knew them, laughed at their jokes. The hospice, she says, did everything they could to keep him feeling like a human being, like himself. At first he resisted their help, but the staff took it in stride and never got angry, says Connie. They let him make as many decisions as he could, about food, about music. "He was very content at last."

During his time at the hospice, spiritual counselor Norma Palazzo arranged for a ceremony with staff members honoring George for his service to the country. This was quite a moving event, Connie recalls. Her husband was bedridden but awake and responsive. Norma read out the words on a certificate: "We pay tribute to you for your military service and for advancing the universal hope of liberty and freedom for all." They thanked him for his service, and shook his hand. This ceremony is one that the hospice performs with every veteran who comes there, part of a program called We Honor Veterans, a collaboration between the National Hospice and Palliative Care Organization and the U.S. Department of Veterans Affairs. The program promotes "respectful inquiry, compassionate listening and grateful acknowledgment" of the veteran's experience.

Norma has a special feeling for the experiences of veterans and their families. Her first husband, a Vietnam veteran, suffered from post-traumatic stress disorder (PTSD) and took his own life. What she and the rest of the staff have learned from preparing the hospice to take part in the We Honor Veterans program is that veterans may have different needs from others at the end of life. Arriving at a hospice is not easy for anyone—a new experience, with new people, a new place, among other difficulties to face. But for veterans, especially those who have seen combat, it may be particularly hard. They may suddenly become hyper-vigilant, "battle ready," unable to trust these new people, uncertain and fearful. This may lead to violent or paranoid behavior. They may not want to be attended by German or Asian caregivers, who remind them of their combat experience.

Hospice workers are trained to go slowly, explain what is going on, try to engage with the dying person in a respectful and collaborative way. They listen carefully to what the veteran has to say, acknowledge his or her experience in the military, express sadness for any suffering, and offer thanks for the service to our country. Some of the old wounds and fears will probably re-emerge, even after a lifetime of pushing them into the background. For old soldiers like George Shally, hospice can bring solace and help assuage some of those wounds.

The Fisher Home has an excellent partner in serving veterans at the end of life—the local Veterans Administration hospital's Kristine Pollard. Kris is a registered nurse who has been working with the V.A. for twenty-three years. As coordinator of the hospice program at the Northampton V.A. Medical Center in Leeds, she follows veterans at the end of life in its long-term care unit as well as in some nursing homes and in their own homes. She is familiar with veterans' special needs, and has known Norma Palazzo for a number of years. Kris sees the Fisher Home as a model for what she would like her own hospice program to be. At the same time, she is an invaluable source of support in helping the hospice take care of veterans.

In a talk to Fisher Home staff and volunteers as they joined the We Honor Veterans program, she pointed out that different wars have produced different psychological effects on those who fought in them. World War II vets, who fought in a "good war," she says, mostly don't want to talk about unpleasant experiences. Vietnam War vets, whose war was not as well supported and whose homecoming she describes as "lousy," may be more willing to talk and express emotion. Different wars also produced different and often unique kinds of injuries and illnesses: tropical diseases and exposure to atomic weapons in World War II; cold injuries, including frostbite, in the Korean War; exposure to Agent Orange in Vietnam; and traumatic brain injuries and amputations in Iraq and Afghanistan.

One of the most helpful things caregivers can do for dying veterans is to sit with them and listen calmly.

Veterans may or may not want to open up about the difficult parts, the "nasty box," says Kris, but if they do, the listener needs to accept what's given, not flinch, not make excuses or try to explain it away. Just tell them you're sorry they've had such a hard experience, that you appreciate their honesty, and thank them for their service, she advises.

Kris is familiar, too, with how medications may or may not work with veterans. Ativan, often used in hospices to alleviate anxiety, may have a "paradoxical" effect, making the ex-soldier even more anxious. When veterans who are accustomed to keeping a tight rein on themselves are given Ativan, they may start reliving the trauma of war and start climbing the walls. If they are competent to make their own decisions, some tough, stoic veterans may refuse all medications and, as she says, "die with their boots on." They need to be granted this choice, she says.

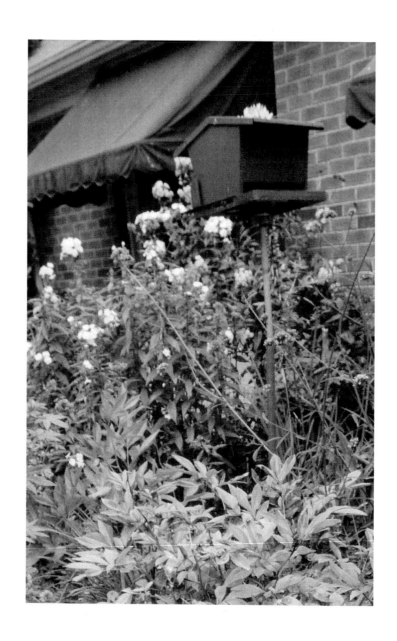

CHAPTER NINETEEN

GERARD STERLING:
A FAMILY'S LONG TRAUMA

MOST OF US WOULD SAY we'd like to die in our sleep, quickly, painlessly. But the slow death, as we've seen for those in hospice care, has its benefits, too, its opportunities for putting things in order, for reconciliations, for coming to terms with the past and with present realities. The slow death is mostly what the Fisher Home deals with. But Dr. Gerard Sterling's death was slow death at its most extreme—a twelve-year slow-motion marathon, a terrible emotional and financial burden that at times left his family in disarray.

Gerard's widow, Lori Beth Sterling, has had to be tough. Dark-haired, fit, intense, she speaks compellingly about the long ordeal of her husband's illness and death. Gerard died at the Fisher Home on May 28, 2013. To keep her family of four children and one grandchild going, Lori Beth works two twenty-four- hour shifts as a nurse paramedic at Armstrong Ambulance, one day in Arlington and one in Burlington, Massachusetts, commuting an hour and a half to each location from her home in Hampden. When her husband was diagnosed with glioblastoma, a deadly brain cancer, their children were fourteen, twelve, nine, and five. All but one of the children now live at home with her.

On the day he first went to the hospital in 2001, Lori Beth was working in Massachusetts and Gerard still had his practice in Florida, commuting north to be with his family once a month. "The plan was for him to work that way for two years, and we'd squirrel away the money from his practice and then he'd move up here and start a new practice," says Lori Beth. Her parents had moved in with them some years earlier.

But their plan was not to be. Gerard had begun having odd symptoms—peripheral vision changes, headaches. Since he'd always had headaches, they could attribute the latest ones to the upsetting fact that his own father was in the hospital. But that wasn't the cause. Says Lori Beth, "I got a call around seven o'clock at night from his manager at Gerard's office in Florida saying something's wrong. He just hadn't been himself that week, and they actually had to drive him home the day before—but nobody had called me then. Now they'd gone over to check on him, and he wouldn't open the door to his apartment. So I called him. His speech was slurred and he was very confused, and I said, 'You need to go to the hospital right now. Open the door and let them come in.' But he wouldn't do it. So I wound up hanging up and calling 911 down there, and I told them just to break the door down." Lori Beth was thirty-nine at the time and Gerard was fifty-two.

The emergency room doctor there was someone she knew, and he told her what was going on. She pauses to think back on that moment. "I don't know," she says, "I've seen people go through the five stages of grief— you know, denial, anger, accepting, the whole thing— but between nine o'clock and three in the morning when we got the CT scan results, I knew in my heart it was a tumor, and I knew it was going to be malignant and that ultimately he was going to die. Literally, there've been bad days and it's gotten me down, but I've been in acceptance ever since his diagnosis. That's the medical part of me. Pretty much everything emotionally that I've gone through since then has just had to do with being overwhelmed with things at times."

She and Gerard had met in an emergency room in Florida, where he was the medical director and she was working for the Broward County Fire Rescue, an air ambulance company. They saw quite a bit of each other in the emergency room, and she was drawn to him. He was thirteen years older, but more importantly, he was mature. "The guys my age in Florida," she explains, "were into big cars, pickup trucks, jet skis, and partying." She liked to have fun, but they were "boys." None of them owned anything; they all rented. Lori Beth had her own paid-for car, had gotten her townhouse—fully furnished—when she was twenty-one. She had money in the bank and was proud of her independence. "Gerard was the physician and I was the nurse and paramedic, but he treated me more like a colleague: 'Hey, what do you think about this?' and 'Do you think this treatment plan is appropriate?' He never looked down on me, and I learned so much." They married a year after they met.

Later, they did exciting, sometimes heroic work, flying Learjets down to the Caribbean, to South America, Europe, and Canada. "We'd repatriate people— patients who were out of the country, people who got sick in another country or people who got sick here and had to go back to their own country." They flew from Haiti to France, a seventeen-hour flight with someone who'd had a motorcycle accident and was a quadriplegic. "If we'd taken him to Miami, which was the closest trauma center, it would have been fifty thousand dollars for his first two days. Instead, by spending the money to send him back to France, it was free medical care." They did that work for three years, and it was great, she says.

Gerard was trained for emergency and critical care. "So" says Lori Beth, "he walked into these little third world nations, and even though they could do things— they had the knowledge—they just didn't have the equipment. So here we show up with basically an ICU unit. We even had dialysis units. We'd stabilize the patient, let the local people help us, and then we'd take the patient to the airport and the whole hospital would come out to see our plane." They had contracts with the military of different countries to pick people up. "We had a family in Orlando whose SUV blew up and there were three burned children, so they called us in to take the children to Shriners in Galveston. We did other stuff in the States all the time, too, stuff like, OK, Grandma's had a stroke and she's recovered but she wants to fly home." They'd take care of people traveling on commercial jets. There they'd be more like a medical escort. The outfit they worked for doesn't exist anymore, but there are dozens of similar ones in Florida, she says.

She misses those days, and misses flying on a helicopter, too, which she did for five years. In addition to her registered nurse's credential, she also has her critical care, flight, and emergency board certifications. After her first son was born, she tried to stay at home but it didn't work, "I loved medicine too much," she says. "I've done so many different things with my nursing and paramedic training—subbed as school nurse, run a field hospital at the Phish concert several years ago on the Vermont–Canada border. It's all been mobile-type nursing. I've never worked in a hospital—don't think I'd want to, either."

After Gerard's initial diagnosis, she brought him

home to Massachusetts. He had one craniotomy, and then a month later they had to do another one, an emergency procedure, because the brain was swelling. They got almost 100 percent of the tumor the first time, says Lori Beth, but it was very aggressive. A month later it was back, the same size.

Meanwhile, having him at home was terrible. One of the things he'd lost, says Lori Beth, was, "let me get the right word for it—the on and off switch. Anything he thought came right out of his mouth, whether it was kind or not." She describes a time when a framed picture of her daughter fell behind the dresser. When Lori Beth's mother went to pick it up, Gerard began screaming at her. She said, "I'm picking it up. The glass has cracked. Do you want me to take it home and get a new frame?" And he shouted, "No! I don't want it!" The child in the picture was sitting right there, says Lori Beth, shaking her head. "I had three kids failing out of school at the same time. I had them in tutoring and stuff, trying to keep them going until I moved him out of the house."

In all, Gerard had two craniotomies, two courses of chemo, a full course of radiation, one of them CT-scan-directed, gamma-knife radiation. And then, she says,

"He actually wanted to go out to California and have some experimental monoclonal antibodies. I stopped him and said, 'First of all, Gerard, it's experimental. Second, it's not covered by insurance. Third, the entire treatment is three or four months. You can't be out there by yourself, and I can't just up and leave the kids and everything with my mom.'" If there had been a chance that he could get something back, she would have said yes, but she knew he was never going to get back his cognitive ability. His old memories were intact but not recent ones. He'd lost the fine motor skills in his hands. He was never going to get his sight back.

"We had some discussions. He really wanted to live, and I don't blame him. He had a prognosis of six months and he got twelve years. The doctors just said, We can't explain it. Be happy with what you have." Of course he wasn't, she says, "and neither would I be."

In December 2002 they initiated hospice care at their home for Gerard, and the day he went into hospice, so did Lori Beth's father. Her father lasted until the end of the following March. He had been very close to her children, getting up at five in the morning to be with them, reading to them, teaching them how to ride their bikes. He was especially important to them after Gerard got sick. Their daughter was eleven, and she was there when her grandfather died, saw him being taken out of the house. Since then, says Lori Beth, the girl has battled depression and anxiety. Lori Beth decided that she didn't want Gerard to have hospice care at home. Aside from the safety issues, she says, "Being relegated to his bedroom downstairs was just as bad as being in a facility."

In 2003 he went to live at Ruth's House, an assisted living facility in Longmeadow, Massachusetts. While he was there, the family would take him out to dinner and to family holidays and birthdays. "We tried to include him in everything," says Lori Beth. "Early on we'd take him to recitals at school and even took a couple of short trips with him. It was a struggle. We had issues when we went out to dinner. People would point at him because he'd lost half his hair. Initially he had a lot of problems with his speech; when he wanted to say something he couldn't find the right words. People thought he was retarded. It was very upsetting."

The length and precariousness of his illness was a constant emotional drain on the family. "We had five times when we thought he was going to die, not counting the last time. I think the kids were already accepting the idea that this is going to happen, but it was so drawn-out that it was kind of like—when?" Her son was in Colorado, and she called him up, and called her nephew who is in the navy, and said: " 'I think this is it; he's seizing every day and he can't talk, he can't walk'—and then two weeks later he'd be fine again. Then a couple of months or a year would go by and we'd do the same thing again." They were all trapped, riding the seesaw. At the end she describes a kind of relief. "Yes, we all cried at the funeral, because we had lost somebody. But it was tears out of: Okay, this journey is finally over. We don't have to have that hanging over our heads constantly now—financially, emotionally."

A couple of weeks before Lori Beth's mother got sick, in 2012, Gerard had some falls that were likely related to seizures, and he went from independent walking to needing a walker. He was then at Ruth's House. By the time of her mother's funeral, he was in a wheelchair, and it took two people to transfer him. "We buried my mom, and I took him home back to Ruth's House, and got him into bed and went downstairs and told them he needed lunch. An hour and a half later they called me and said he was seizing up a storm. That was the last thing—he never got out of bed again. It took us a week to get him up to Amherst with all the insurance junk."

After that, Gerard kept asking his wife, "What can I do to make this go faster?" And the only thing she could say was, "Do like my mom did and stop eating. There's nothing else legally we can do." At the very end he did just that, started refusing food. But before that, at Ruth's House and afterward at the Fisher Home, he ate the same meals every day: two egg whites scrambled, orange juice and toast in the morning, tuna sandwich at lunch, and a salad at night—a regular ritual. When the family took him out for a birthday to a Chinese restaurant, he'd eat a whole platter of different food. Then, as soon as he went back, he only wanted those same three meals.

Lori Beth has seen what she thinks of as bad end-of-life care. When her mother was in a nursing home that also provided hospice care, she thought the hospice providers were great, but they weren't there all the time. She was unhappy with the facility's nurses, who were not hospice trained. "Their attitude was: Feed 'em, clean 'em, turn 'em." They kept bringing her mother food even though she couldn't eat. "Their idea is to get people well and go home. I had to keep reminding them: She's not going home."

About her experience at the Fisher Home, she has only positive things to say. "Never went in there and found him in a state I would be upset with. They always kept me abreast of everything that was going on, included me in all the care plans, respected our wishes, worked with me when the insurance companies were cutting Gerard off."

Before that, she says, she'd had to fight with nurses and doctors. As a seasoned medical professional, she was usually able to prevail. At one point when Gerard was at Ruth's House, he fell and broke his orbit, the bone around the eye socket. At this point, he already had a Do Not Resuscitate order. Says Lori Beth, "He'd had a small bleed and they wanted to watch him overnight in the hospital. And the nurse came in and said: I have to start an IV. And I said, 'Gerard, do you want an IV?' And he said no. And I said to the nurse, 'He doesn't want one.' 'Well, you have to have one.' 'Why?' 'Because he's being admitted.' And I said, 'Well, is he going to be kept NPO (nothing by mouth)?' 'No.' 'Is he going to get IV antibiotics?' 'No.' 'Is he getting IV pain meds?' 'No.' 'Well then, you don't need it.' 'Well, we have to have it if something happens.' 'If something happens he has a DNR. He doesn't want anything done if something happens.' " Lori Beth went and got the doctor, who agreed with what she and her husband were saying.

At that point the nurse went out and found another nurse. The first nurse wouldn't take care of him, saying, "DNR doesn't mean do not treat." Lori Beth agreed, then asked, "Does he have something for pain?" Yes, orders for Percoset, by mouth. "So," Lori Beth said, "he doesn't need or want an IV."

She describes a similar argument with a doctor who wanted to do all kinds of tests. She said, " 'Doctor, do what you feel you have to do to protect yourself, but when you rack up a big bill for the insurance for someone who doesn't want anything done and isn't going to do anything, then what is going on here?' " Insurance companies had to be battled as well. She says she might still have to pay $13,000 out of pocket. The last insurance company said they'd pay for six months and only paid for five. She's on her second appeal.

There were no battles at the Fisher Home. Everybody was helpful, says Lori Beth—"Donna Sarro in the financial office; Lucy the nurse, she was a doll; Ilsa was a sweetheart." She trusted the people there, knew

Gerard was taken care of and that they'd follow the care plan. She didn't have the feeling that she had to be there every minute to intercede for him. "If I called, they'd say, 'Just call in the middle of the night if you need to know.'" She was out of town when Gerard died, two weeks after they had expected. "I'd put off so many things in my life because, well—what if?" She had talked to the people at the Fisher Home, and they said, "'Just go. We'll keep you informed.' In the end he really didn't know if you were there or not. They gave me permission to go without feeling bad about it."

At least, says Lori Beth, "He got to see the kids grow up and see what kind of people they were going to be."

Interesting conversation with the
wife of E. She is a round-faced,
chipper woman, humorous and down-to-
earth, lives on her own in one of the
western Massachusetts hill towns. She
has brought him here during the winter because she didn't think she
could keep him at home, and knew it
would be hard to get caregivers into
the hills in snow and ice. She said
she did her grieving when she had to
bring him here, and that it isn't so
bad now. She is here often, sees this
place as her second home.

A conversation with Ilsa about how
people need to be better educated
about hospice. I mention my contact
with a friend who is now under hospice
care at home in Northampton. How can
we take the stigma, as it were, the
reluctance, off hospice? Make it not
feel like a death sentence. First, I
guess, you have to accept the fact of
a terminal status--your own.

N. has "graduated," not been recertified, and has gone home with her
daughter, who came by with two plates
of mini-cream puffs. She also left a
letter of thanks, similar to others
posted on a bulletin board in the
hallway near the kitchen.

"You took my mom into your home and
into your hearts at the most vulnera-
ble of times. For six months, you
attended to her with gentle kindness
as she teetered precariously between
this world and the next. With tender-
ness, you brought sanctity to the
mundane tasks of the washing, feeding
and changing my mom. With generosity,
you brought your prayers, your reading, and your wonderful music to her
bedside."

***

I. is now dying--"actively," and her
two daughters are sitting vigil. There
is a son, but he's at a distance and
having more trouble bringing himself
here. It's a problem for men, I say,
don't you think? They agree. Maybe
they're more used to keeping their
emotions inside, so find them hard to
deal with when they come to the surface? The daughters seem pleased to
have someone else to talk to.

Volunteer George Maston has been
busy in the kitchen making breakfast.
He filled me in on various new people,
including one elderly gent, R., who
is French, and who had been imprisoned
in France with his family during World

War II. I meet his family and hope to
learn more. R. likes to speak French.
I will try.

***

A quiet day. Only four patients. I
water the potted plants outside the
entries, then talk briefly with E., a
new resident, out in the geri-chair,
a recliner on wheels, with his partner. It is his birthday. They are sitting on the little porch near the
entrance, she bent over his arm. They
evidently "married" each other yesterday, without benefit of intermediary,
having already been spiritually married for years. He wears a wool hat,
is somewhat unshaven, has bright blue
eyes, as does she. He is said to have
a strong spiritual practice, and is
holding some prayer beads. His room is
filled with icons of various sorts,
mostly from Eastern sources, mandalas,
Buddhas, plus Native American sand
paintings.

***

Today, the annual potluck memorial
picnic, a great success. About forty
families show up, probably seventy-five
people, milling about, giving and

getting hugs. I had worried about
Susan Sachs, who with her sister Linda
made a memorial garden that had become
quite ragged looking. Joan Roach and I
worked on it to restore its heart
shape and added new colorful plants. I
had put a small frog statue at the top
of the heart, but Joan decided it
wasn't respectful enough, so I put the
frog in the birdbath and brought one of
my bigger shells--a conch--from home
and put it where the frog had been.
Susan is delighted. We talk about her
father and his quirks. Howard had made
quite a fuss about food at the end, and
she reminds me that he ate nothing but
matzos with raspberry jam, and sent it
back if the jam was too close to the
edge and got on his fingers.

Board member Father Bill Hamilton
gives an invocation describing his own
near-death experience in a car crash.
I am a little nervous about how religious this is going to be. We are so
vigilant about being spiritually nonspecific, nondenominational. But he is
careful, remaining mostly humorous and
folksy.

After he speaks, the names of the
people who died during the year are
read by a number of staff and

volunteers, a moving roll call. Then
Norma invites all the little kids to
the front and has them open a box
that comes from the local butterfly
conservatory. They release about
twenty butterflies, with one ,of them
magically staying on the arm of one
of the little girls, seemingly not
wanting to fly away.

***

Lucy says E. is looking for company,
so I stop by. Beth has been going
through a family photo album with him,
so I sit at the foot of his bed and
start looking, too. He tells me in
some detail about his past. He'd run
away from home as a teen and joined
a hippie commune, eventually married.
He'd managed a secondhand, "collect-
ibles" shop in California. Pictures
of him as a young adult show a strong,
confident-looking physical presence
building houses, dealing with children.
     He wears a wool hat, and much of
the time his eyes are partly shut or
gazing at the ceiling. I am not sure
how close to sleep he is, so stop
talking. He starts up again, talking
about how this "thing"--rectal

cancer--had dropped onto him, and how
it has changed his life, in some ways
for the better. A son who had been
estranged is back in touch and has
wept with him. After a while, E. tells
me he thinks I seem very spiritual.
Oh, I say, what makes you say that?
Just a feeling, he says. He asks me
about my spiritual life, and I say
that I was a Catholic in my youth, but
no longer take part in any organized
set of beliefs. I believe in decency,
in honesty, in love, in work. He says
he wishes he had met me sooner. I say
I will come back and see him. He has
made it clear to the staff that he is
"searching" for a spiritual home. He
seems quite a lost soul to me.

***

E. died a few days after our conversation. Beth tells me about the incident of the cardinal. Had I heard? It
seems that after his father's death
E.'s son, the one who had been
estranged, went to Puffer's Pond, a
local watering hole, for a swim and to
think about things. On his way back,
he saw a cardinal in the road. He

stopped and picked it up to keep it
safe. When he got to the hospice he
let it go, but it didn't fly away. Beth
then saw it sitting on top of her car.
She felt it was a sign of some sort.

***

On my way out, I pick up my old copy
of Sherlock Holmes, which I find on a
shelf in the hall. Gerard is gone, and
there is another copy, much bigger and
newer, on the same shelf. I got lucky
when I discovered Gerard's love for
those stories.

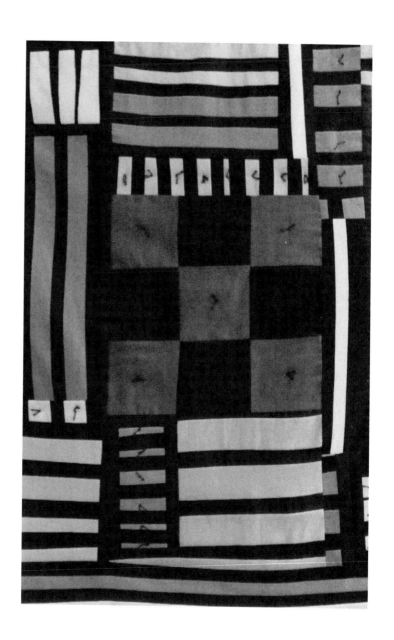

CHAPTER TWENTY

MAXINE STEIN:
MAKING ORDER,
REACHING OUT

I N THE TIME SINCE MAXINE ARRIVED, in January 2013, she has shown herself to be an agent of change, both physically and organizationally— getting rid of the excess stuff that had accumulated in the building and its storage rooms, cupboards, and drawers. At the same time she has worked to clear out the unhelpful habits of a workplace that had been without a leader for over a year. She has made space, both inside the building and inside the organization, so that people can function better.

In mid-May, a volunteer cleanup day was scheduled, to get rid of stuff that was no longer functional or needed. Volunteers and staff filled a huge dumpster with old cabinets, broken lamps and chairs, and other debris that had piled up indoors and out. Cleaning out the place, Maxine says, was for her "symbolic of getting the house in order."

The new director has a professional air. Except when helping to fill up a dumpster, she dresses in chic, tailored outfits and high-heeled shoes, and is always perfectly put together. She has a knack of seeing what needs to be done and doing it without encroaching on other people's turf. Stopping in the kitchen to talk with the granddaughters of one of the residents, she engages them in an animated conversation about Israel, where they are living, and where Maxine's stepchildren live. She takes her time with these visitors, but it is clear that she won't neglect her next task.

When she arrived at the Fisher Home, she immediately went to work reorganizing the staff's physical environment. The nurses' office, where the clinical director has her desk and where all the medical records are kept, was moved to the opposite end of the building, closer to the nurses' station. Two offices were carved out of a larger one, and now house Maxine and her invaluable administrative assistant, Karen Howery. A conference room was created out of an underused library. Updated office equipment and supplies were tucked neatly into a former storage closet. Other physical changes are making it easier for people to have space, boundaries, privacy, and a sense of professionalism.

These four elements are also crucial to the changes Maxine saw as needing to be made in how the staff communicates with one another. Without those anchors, she believes, you wind up with a general lack of trust. When she arrived, she found confusion—one person saying one thing, another saying something different. It was like the old children's game of "telephone," she says. Information was passed from person to person, getting changed and distorted along the way. It wasn't clear who was in charge, how decisions got made. People were asking, "Who can we listen to? Who can we believe?" Things needed to be sorted out, she says, questions answered: "Is this a true democracy, or is there a hierarchy? Do we decide by consensus? What decisions can be made by consensus and what can't?" What she saw, put tactfully, was a "less established organizational structure."

To firm up that structure, she has worked to set up clearer lines of communication. If it's a nursing question, don't come to Maxine. That has to go through clinical director Kathy Curtis. If it's about nursing assistants, we need to include Jenn Messinger in the conversation. Those things seem automatic to her as executive director, but she's found that they are very much appreciated here. She's been sending out memos to the staff, "sharing what we're doing"—another no-brainer, she says. Why *wouldn't* she do that? "My hope is just to help the hospice run better and better, to make people working here feel good and to like how it's being done."

All that is on the inside of the hospice. But Maxine also wants the world to know "what a premiere place this is, a jewel of western Massachusetts, a treasure, an incredible resource." She's clear that good work is being done by other local hospice programs, but she wants people to think first of the Fisher Home when they want a combined community and inpatient program staffed by people who are "truly centered and know what they're doing." These aspects of the Fisher Home already exist, but she wants to add more—speakers for the community, educational resources about death and dying.

For this vision to become a reality, Maxine needs better marketing and fund-raising. Work is being done to improve the hospice's website, and they're doing some "thoughtful recruiting" on the hospice's board, replacing people who are cycling off. "We need high visibility; we need philanthropy," she says. For that she needs people with deep connections to the community, not just deep pockets. "The Valley needs to own this place, to say, 'This is ours. This is a resource that we all need, and we're going to take care of it and support it.' " She wants to make sure that it not only continues but also grows. She's been meeting with fund-raising groups to see that the Fisher Home is on their radar, and to get advice about donors and possible grants. In addition, she and Kathy Curtis have been on the road, talking with marketing people from different medical groups. The two of them met recently with providers from a large local group: "A lot of them didn't know about our community service," the fact that the Fisher Home also provides hospice service in people's homes. "That's the secret." That secret obviously needs to get out. One key to this is a new hire, community nurse Monica Susskind, who has been working to expand the number of patients the hospice cares for in their homes, with the understanding that they can move to the hospice residence if and when they need to.

Maxine's former work experience makes her well qualified for this job. She has been a fund-raiser, a marketer, and an executive director, with much of her time spent in medical and human services organizations, including four years as program director at a hospice in Saint Louis, Missouri. She holds a master's in social work, has headed a national organization for the prevention of child sexual abuse, and was executive director of the National Ovarian Cancer Coalition. Her most recent job was as director of development for the Yiddish Book Center in Amherst. She knows the philanthropic landscape of this area well. Along with that, she has what Norma Palazzo calls "a hospice heart," the understanding and sympathy needed to provide humane options for the end of life.

Says Maxine, "There just aren't that many of us"— independently run, freestanding hospices that also offer home care. Most freestanding hospices are connected to larger institutions—hospitals, home nursing, and home hospice organizations. Maxine has been meeting with other hospice organizations, and they talk about the luxury of a residential hospice. Often the residential hospice is a loss leader to a larger institution, but, she says, it's a feather in their cap to have the residence. Since the Fisher Home is on its own, "We don't have that luxury." And there's no plan to affiliate with a larger organization, "certainly not in my vision," Maxine says, nor in the board's.

So the challenges reside in the business model, in money. Because the Fisher Home is so dependent on the home's census—the number of residents at any given time—it is financially unstable. "People on the outside say, Well, you have a waiting list— which is true, but it doesn't work that way in hospice," she explains. You may have a long waiting list, but at the moment when people need a residential hospice, if there's not a space, they either stay where they are, move somewhere else that's permanent, or die. "It's the kind of service that when you need it, you need it now."

For the moment, there will be no more physical changes. "I've run out of money," she says. "If someone came and said, 'I'd like to give you thirty thousand dollars to redo the kitchen, I'd be thrilled." Even before that happened, if it were possible, another space she'd like to add is a counseling room. It could be a small room—a quiet space away from the center of things, away from the patients, the call bells, away from the nursing staff and the comings and goings in the hall— someplace you could have an undisturbed confidential conversation.

Many other hoped-for enhancements will have to wait—for instance a memorial garden. Much as Maxine would like to have it, it's not on her priority list; there are just too many other things that need taking care of: "It's already overwhelming, a huge piece of property. We own it and don't have a landlord to fix the driveway and the potholes." Suggestions are nice, says Maxine, but it's a lot more than doing something pretty. It's all about maintenance. Systems are fragile in an old building. "I feel like the poor young married couple. Everytime something breaks, it throws off your finances."

But for the Fisher Home, finances are linked to a place in the community consciousness, something that hasn't happened enough—not yet, anyway. Not enough people know about this wonderful place, Maxine says, and she plans to change that.

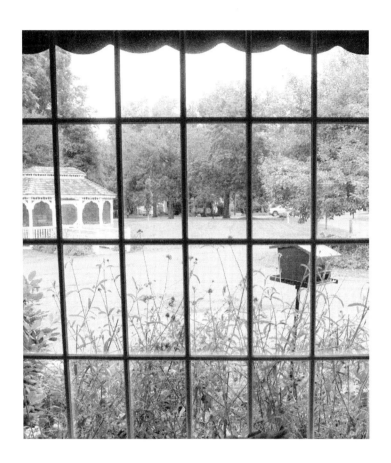

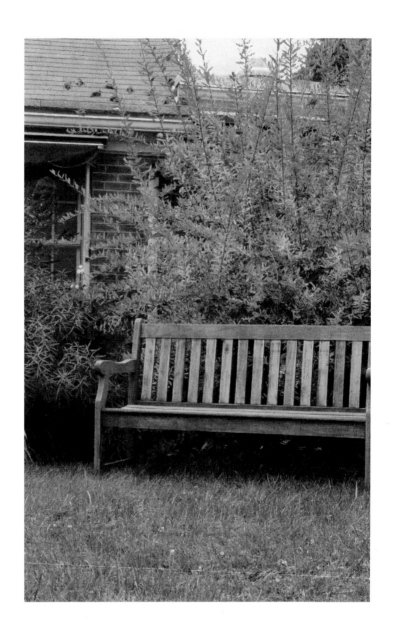

CHAPTER TWENTY-ONE

OVERNIGHT:
KEEPING WATCH

USUALLY I'M AT THE HOSPICE during the day, so I know what it looks and sounds like, but I've been curious about the night shift, so I ask to stay over for one. Although the shift starts at midnight, Bob Nelson, the nurse, and June Bishop, the aide, get there a good half hour early. They make a good team. Bob is thorough, patient, professorial, an excellent person for an observer to follow since he describes everything he's doing and why he's doing it. June is more intuitive, quick to see a resident's needs, ready to stroke a forehead, ask "How're you doin', sweetheart?," then call Bob in to administer pain medication or help move someone. They turn bedridden people every two hours, and put pillows behind one woman's back. Her spine is beginning to show signs of redness, the precursor of a worrisome but preventable bedsore. They listen for sounds, mostly the sounds of breathing during this nighttime shift, but what they really attend to are changes of any sort.

The lights are on all over the building's hallways. In fact, there seems to be more light than in the daytime. Most residents' rooms have some sort of gentle light burning, and most people are sleeping soundly. This way the staff can look in and see what's happening. It is a busier night than usual, because one resident is having a lot of pain, this time in his chest. He has bladder cancer as well as a broken hip and collarbone from a fall that occurred before he came here. In addition, several of the residents seem to be actively dying, as it's called.

In one of the rooms there is an aide from an agency

who has been hired to watch over the husband of K., one of the residents. K. is dying of cancer, and her husband is staying with her, sleeping on a cot in the room. The Fisher Home tries to make this arrangement available to any relative who wants to stay with the dying person, but there had been a special problem here because the husband has dementia, and although he is mostly peaceful and amenable, he tends to wander. The hospice administration made it clear to the family that he could stay only if he had his own attendant to keep track of him. So there are always three people in this room—the resident in a hospital bed, the spouse on a cot, and the aide in a reclining chair.

The first order of business is for Bob to "get report" from the nurse who is finishing her 4 p.m. to midnight shift. They sit at a table in the conference room. There are no visitors or bustle at this hour, so the door can remain open, as it would not during the day. Outside are only the trilling of peepers and other sounds of a late spring night, along with occasional traffic on the road far down the driveway. Checking her own written notes, the afternoon nurse goes through the rooms in numerical order, describing each resident's condition, what changes occurred, how much food was eaten, how much and what kind of "output"—bowel and urine—there had been, what medications were given in what dosages and at what times. Levels of pain and other discomfort are registered, along with any action, medicinal and otherwise, to alleviate them. Bob listens, asking questions and taking his own notes from hers. His notes are color-coded: red for the notes he keeps all day, black for the permanent ones at the end of the shift.

One incident involves K., who had been having some nausea but lately had been feeling better. In the afternoon she was visited by a friend, who had given her a back rub, which she had enjoyed. But immediately afterward, K. began to vomit again and was very distressed. Medications had been administered, and the vomiting subsided. Was the back rub the cause of the upset? Well intentioned, but perhaps too stimulating? they wonder. As they go through the notes on different residents, they discuss the needs and wishes of their families but mainly place their emphasis on the patients' wishes. If they are responsive, residents are always asked whether they want more pain medication, something for their nausea, something to eat or drink, company or not.

When they finish exchanging information, the afternoon nurse goes to the nurses' station and begins filling out the forms that will be her official notes for the day. She will be here for another hour and a half working on them.

Meanwhile, in the kitchen, June, who hates to be idle, has been cleaning every surface with disinfecting cloths and is preparing a chocolate Bundt cake, which she'll frost with chocolate icing and colored sprinkles, then put out in the dining room for general enjoyment. She has already checked all the rooms to see what needs to be done. She'll do this throughout her shift, talking to people who are awake to see if they are comfortable, responding to the bells that residents ring if they want help going to the bathroom, need to complain of pain, or simply want company.

Z. is sleeping but seems restless, and is in an odd position with her arm extended over her head, making random jerky motions. Is this a sign of some change? June asks Bob. They check her pulse, her temperature. Nothing different in her vital signs; they'll keep an eye on her. The resident with chest pain gets some extra medication. They check the morphine pump of a woman who has been making moaning sounds. They look to see if anyone needs to have incontinence briefs changed. They again turn the people who need to be turned, talking to them gently as they do so. Staff members are careful not to speak as though the dying person were not in the room. Residents are addressed directly and told what's happening: "Hello, Jim, we're here to turn you. Can you settle back a little? That's good. We're going to pull you up in the bed and straighten out this bedding so you can be more comfortable. Now we're going to put these pillows behind your back. How's that? Better? Good." Hearing, we are told, is the last of the senses to leave a dying person.

Around 4 a.m. it begins to get light, and the birds are making quite a racket. June takes a short break outside—she's a smoker—after delivering the trash and recyclables to the plastic containers in the garage, then putting them out for the morning's pickup.

Z. has been having a difficult night, and Bob predicts that she may not survive until morning. But she is scheduled for a bed bath at 6 a.m., before breakfast preparations begin. For the past few days Z. has needed an oxygen mask, and she's now fighting hard to breathe,

the cavities next to her thin collarbone sucking in with each inhalation. June has sat with her whenever she's had a free moment, talking to her and stroking her arm and forehead. "It's okay, sweetheart," she says. "It's okay." Z. cannot respond. She has not spoken in days. The TV in her room is set to a channel that plays light classical music around the clock, Z.'s choice. The volume is set very low tonight. Around 6 a.m., Jane goes in to begin the bed bath, closing the door for the sake of modesty. A few minutes later she comes out. Z. is gone. The difficult breathing is over.

Z. has been at the hospice for ten months, bedridden the whole time, with breast cancer that has invaded much of the rest of her body. An eye and her nose are disfigured by this disease. She is eighty-seven, a single woman. There are a couple of nieces, one of whom lives in New England, a few hours away, the other in Florida. When I've been at the hospice during her stay here, I've never encountered a relative or friend. Yet Z. has been a sweet, if mostly a passive, presence. When she arrived, she was chatty, showed some sparks of humor, enjoyed being read to, enjoyed especially singing a slightly off-color song that began: "Oh, the monkey curled his tail around the flagpole /

And showed his asshole to the crowd." She came from a Catholic family, never married, outlived her siblings, and had lived alone in Springfield, where she'd worked as a secretary. After one of the big storms that damaged the area, she was brought to the hospice.

I had occasionally read to her and often fed her, held her hand and talked to her when she wailed, which she sometimes did for no obvious reason, except for the fact that she was alone in a place where she was living out her last days. There was one volunteer who had developed a real relationship with her. Everyone agreed that she was sweet, and she had certainly turned out to have a strong hold on life.

After he has taken his stethoscope and "pronounced" Z.'s death, Bob calls the niece who lives closest. She asks that we gather up all the family photographs, without their frames, and Z.'s rosaries. There are four of these. There are not a lot of other possessions—a few cheerful birthday and Mother's Day cards pinned to the wall. Z.'s clothing is to be donated to the hospice, where June says it will be welcome, since it is in good condition and includes bathrobes and gowns that open up and are easy to put on. Bob calls the funeral home in Springfield where arrangements are already in place. Its van will be getting here in an hour or so.

The shift is ending, and Bob prepares his notes to give report to Matt, the nurse who will be arriving at 7:30 for the 8 a.m. to 4 p.m. shift.

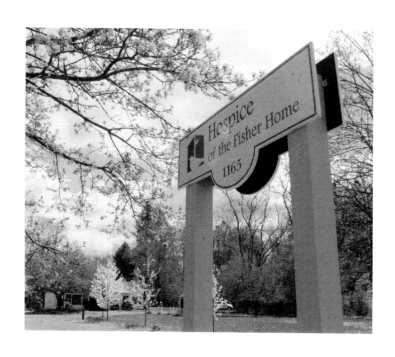

Epilogue
A LOGO

D URING MAXINE STEIN'S FIRST YEAR
as director of the Fisher Home, she and the
board decided to revisit the hospice's logo,
the defining image that appears on its letterhead, bro-
chure, and website. They wanted to create a new image
for the organization, one that showed its dual nature as
a provider of both home and residential hospice care.
Working with a designer, they asked themselves what
was unique about the place, and settled on a design of
a bird superimposed on a two-part birdhouse. While
offering a symbolic representation of the organization's
twin services, the design also presents a more literal
representation, a birdhouse and a generic New England
bird that might come to the feeder outside each patient's
window at the hospice residence.

I am not normally a believer in the power of logos, especially for organizations that care for the spirit as well as the body, but this one has grown on me. Along with being attractive, it strikes me as having a resonance beyond its original intent. In my experience with staff, patients, and families at the hospice, birds and other beautiful winged beings have often come to represent something beyond life and death. In one account, a flock of birds came to a feeder just after a resident's life ended. In another, the son of a resident who had recently died rescued a bird from traffic, and the bird remained at the hospice for several days. On a different occasion, hawks swooped down on the cars of relatives of a departed resident. At the memorial picnic, one of the freed butterflies stayed to perch peacefully on a child's arm. These events were meaningful to the people who observed them, giving them a sense of being in touch in a special way with someone who had gone from this life.

Evidently something about birds reminds us of our mortality and the hope of an afterlife. Like the human spirit or soul, perhaps, they are fragile but strong; they can do things that the human frame cannot—fly, soar, ride the wind. There are religions in which the image of the bird depicts spirituality itself, an emblem of the soul or the holy spirit. In some traditions, a window is opened after a person dies to let the soul fly out, as if it were a caged bird that had now been set free. In a piece of writing that I keep coming back to, the Venerable Bede, an eighth-century English monk, compares the fleetingness of human life to a bird flying through a banquet hall. The monk addresses his king:

> When compared with the stretch of time unknown to us, O king, the present life of men on earth is like the flight of a single sparrow through the hall where, in winter, you sit with your captains and ministers. Entering at one door and leaving by another, while it is inside it is untouched by the wintry storm; but this brief interval of calm is over in a moment, and it returns to the winter whence it came, vanishing from your sight. Man's life is similar; and of what follows it, or what went before, we are utterly ignorant.[*]

I find this short speech moving and evocative. The metaphor of human life as a brief passage between two

---

[*] D. J. Enright, ed., *The Oxford Book of Death* (Oxford: Oxford University Press, 1983), 2.

unknowns, with the analogy of the bird moving through a temporary place of warmth and companionship, feels just right to me. I am especially comfortable with its tone of restraint, its lack of certainty about what comes before or after.

The vocabulary of hospice often refers to the end of life as part of a journey, a passage—like the bird's through the banquet hall. In fact, a common synonym for dying is "passing away," or simply "passing." A small, independent, nonprofit hospice cannot remove the mystery from that passage, but it offers a model for how to complete the journey in the company of thoughtful, compassionate, and skilled people, with the warmth, comfort, and companionship we hope to find in the rest of our lives. At the Hospice of the Fisher Home, it is understood that the work of helping people die in peace requires many hands.

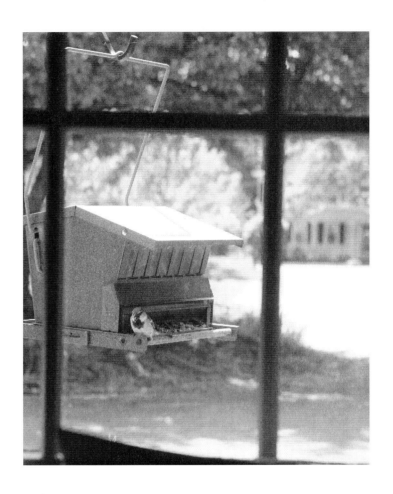

ACKNOWLEDGMENTS

Chris Jerome encouraged, chastened, pruned, and edited my writing all the way along. James McDonald turned my words into a handsome book. Mickey Rathbun and Kim Townsend were helpful readers. And Bill Pritchard, as always, set an example of how things get written.

A different version of Chapter 18, "Veterans: Bringing Them Home," appeared in the *Daily Hampshire Gazette*, Northampton, Massachusetts.

BOOKS CONSULTED

My book relies primarily on observations and interviews, but it draws also from my readings on death and dying, on the history and practice of hospice, on old age, and on the state of medicine in this country. This list covers only the books I found especially useful; it does not include newspaper or magazine articles. The books are listed in order of their importance to me.

Clendinen, Dudley. *A Place Called Canterbury*
(New York: Viking, 2008).
This book about a retirement home in Florida, its inhabitants and staff, served as a model for the book I was hoping to write, with its combination of engagement and detachment. Clendinen later wrote a moving article in the *New York Times Magazine* about facing his own impending death from amyotrophic lateral sclerosis (ALS). He died in 2012.

Barnes, Julian. *Nothing to Be Frightened Of*
(New York: Knopf, 2009).
A wonderfully humane and witty memoir exploring different possible attitudes toward death.

Stoddard, Sandol. *The Hospice Movement: A Better Way of Caring for the Dying* (New York: Vintage, 1992).
A definitive account of the founding, growth, and philosophy of hospice.

Byock, Ira. *Dying Well: Peace and Possibilities at the End of Life* (New York: Riverhead, 1997).
Using case histories, Byock, a hospice doctor, argues for allowing the end of life to be both meaningful and pain-free.

Kiernan, Stephen P. *Last Rights: Rescuing the End of Life from the Medical System* (New York: St. Martin's, 2006).
A well-researched, readable book describing how resistant to change our acute-care system has been, and the cost of that resistance, both in money and misery.

Doka, Kenneth J., Jennings, Bruce, and Corr, Charles A., eds. *Ethical Dilemmas at the End of Life* (Washington, DC: Hospice Foundation of America, 2005).
Essays considering philosophical, religious, cultural, medical, and ideological perspectives on the care of the dying.

Kübler-Ross, Elisabeth. *On Death and Dying; Questions and Answers on Death and Dying; On Life after Death* (New York: Quality Paperback Book Club, 2002).
This book's first section, aimed at confronting society's fear of death, famously describes the five stages people go through when they learn they are dying. It was first published in this country in 1969.

Wolff, Sara S. *Vital Aging: Seven Years of Building Community and Enhancing Health* (Amherst, MA: Levellers, 2010).
Sara Wolff, who died at the Fisher Home, had been as clear-eyed about aging as she was about her own death.

Sachs, Howard. *Skydiving Into Medical School and Other Adventures from the Slums of New York to the Himalayas: A Memoir by Howard Sachs Ph.D., M.D.* (Big Story Productions, 2011).
An edited version of the blog kept by Howard Sachs and published a few months before his death at the Fisher Home. The title speaks for itself.

The Way to Go was designed
by James McDonald
of The Impress Group,
Northampton, Massachusetts.
JAMESMCDONALDBOOKS.COM
The text is set in Stickley 12/18.